Ann has D

Sheila Hollins, Noë ...kman
and Ruth Eley
illustrated by Lisa Kopper

Beyond Words

1

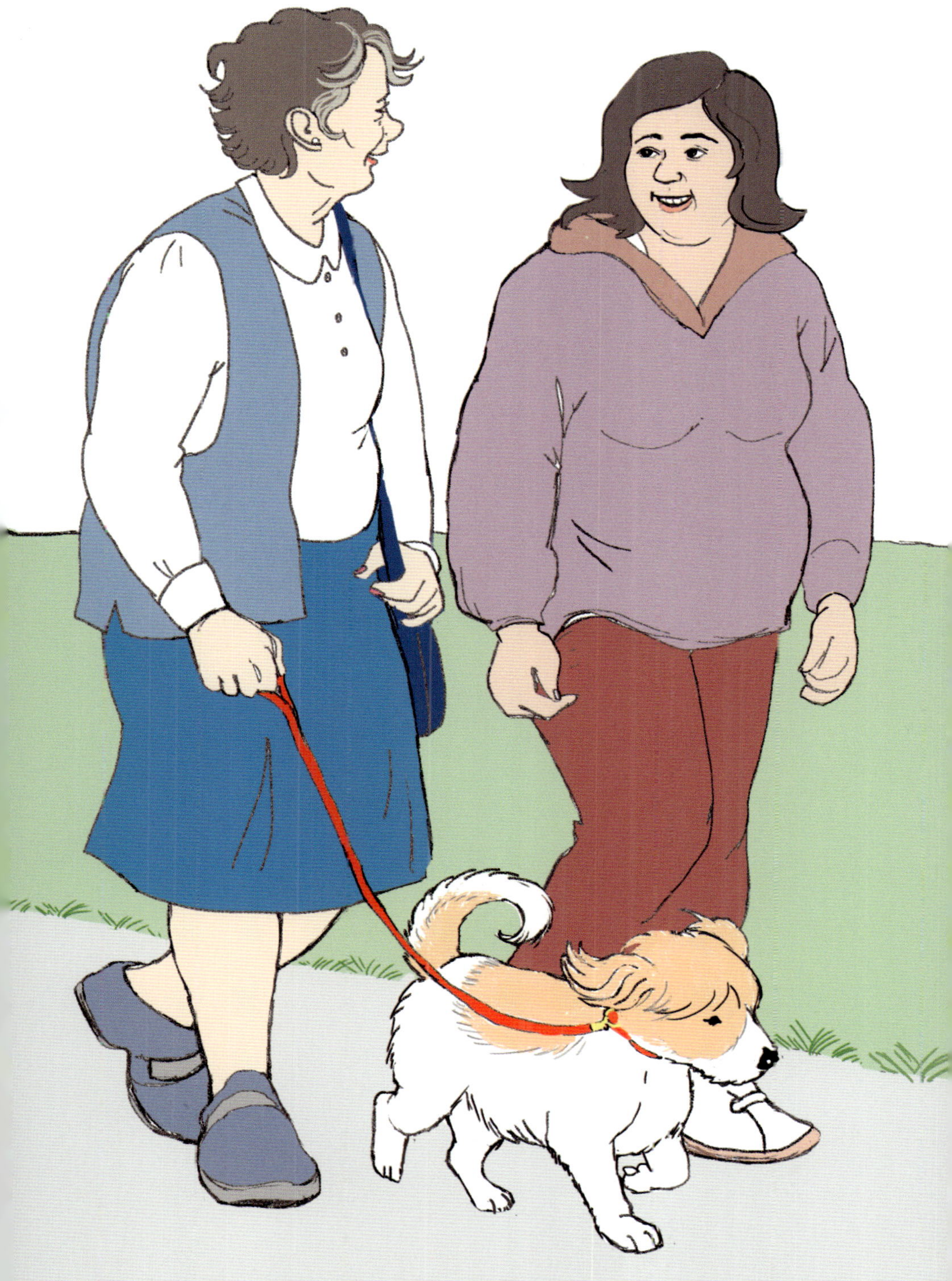

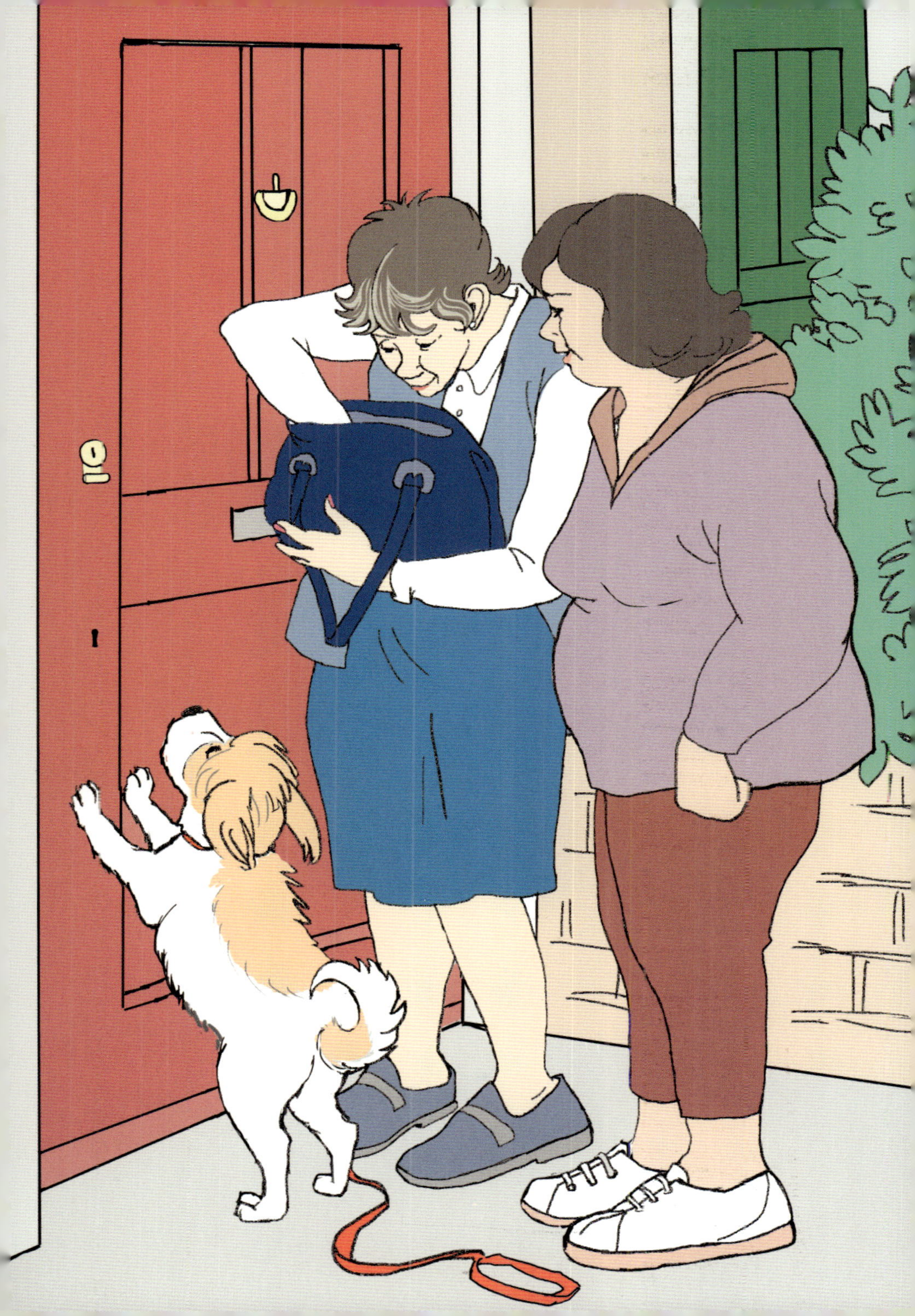

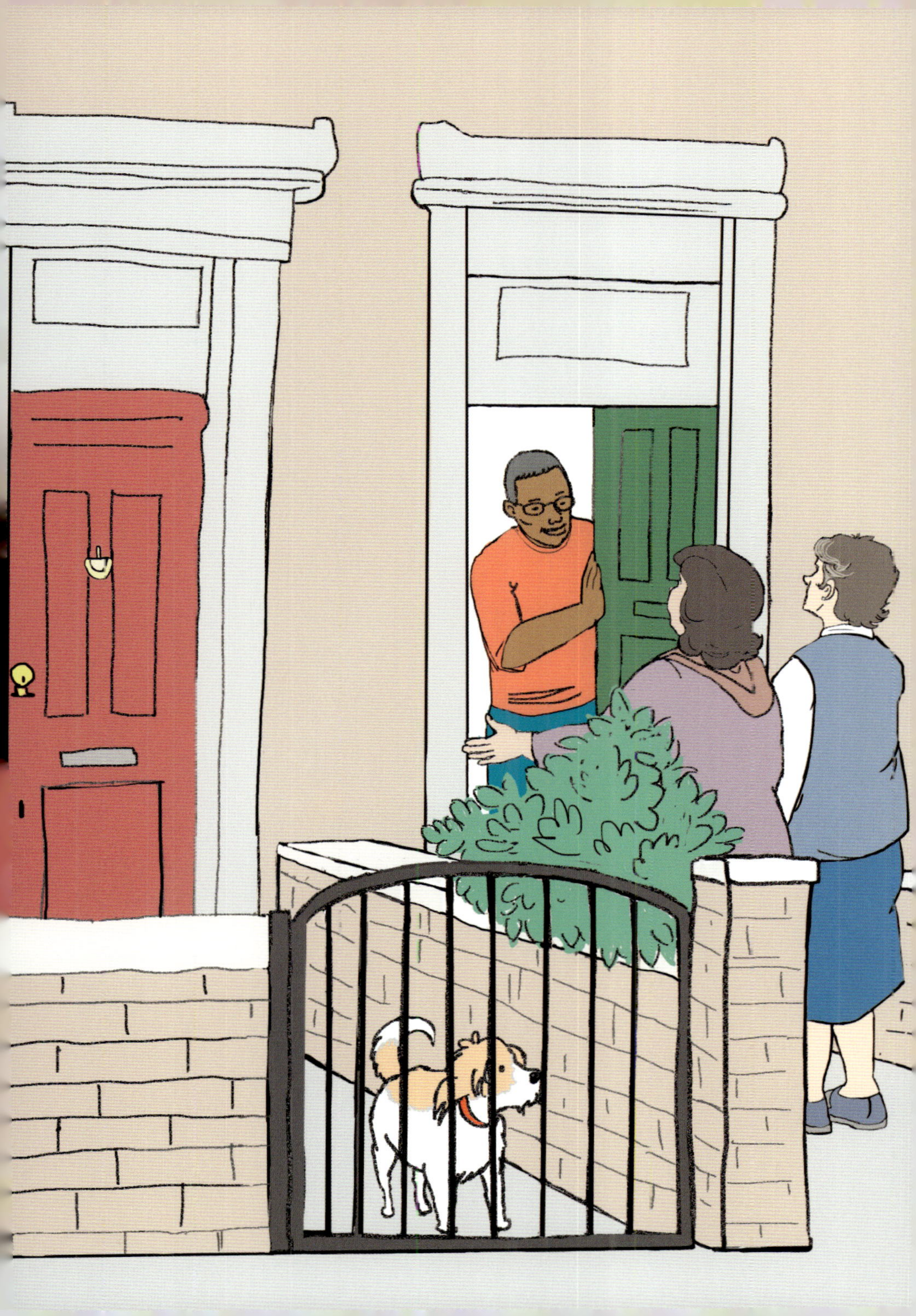

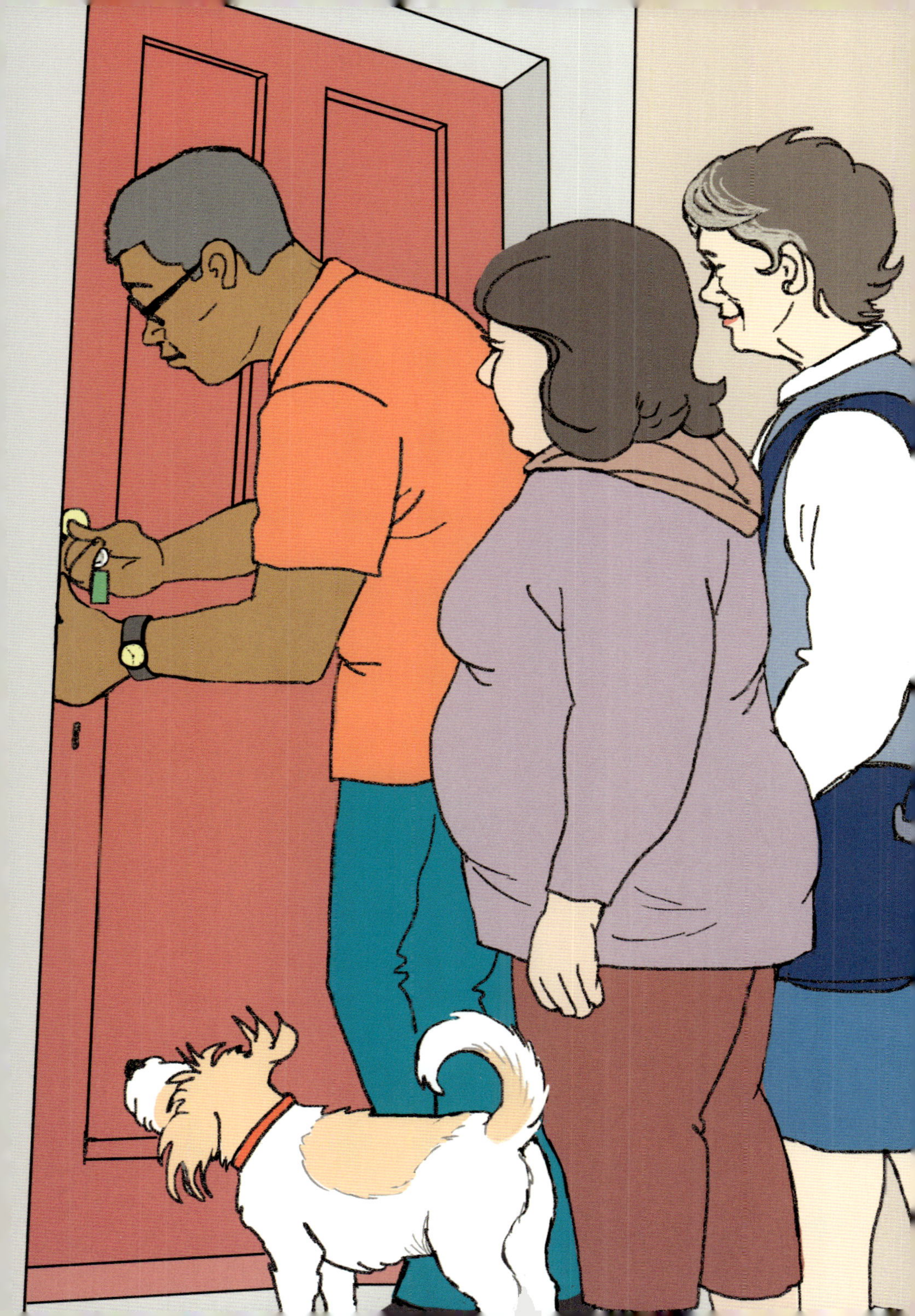

5

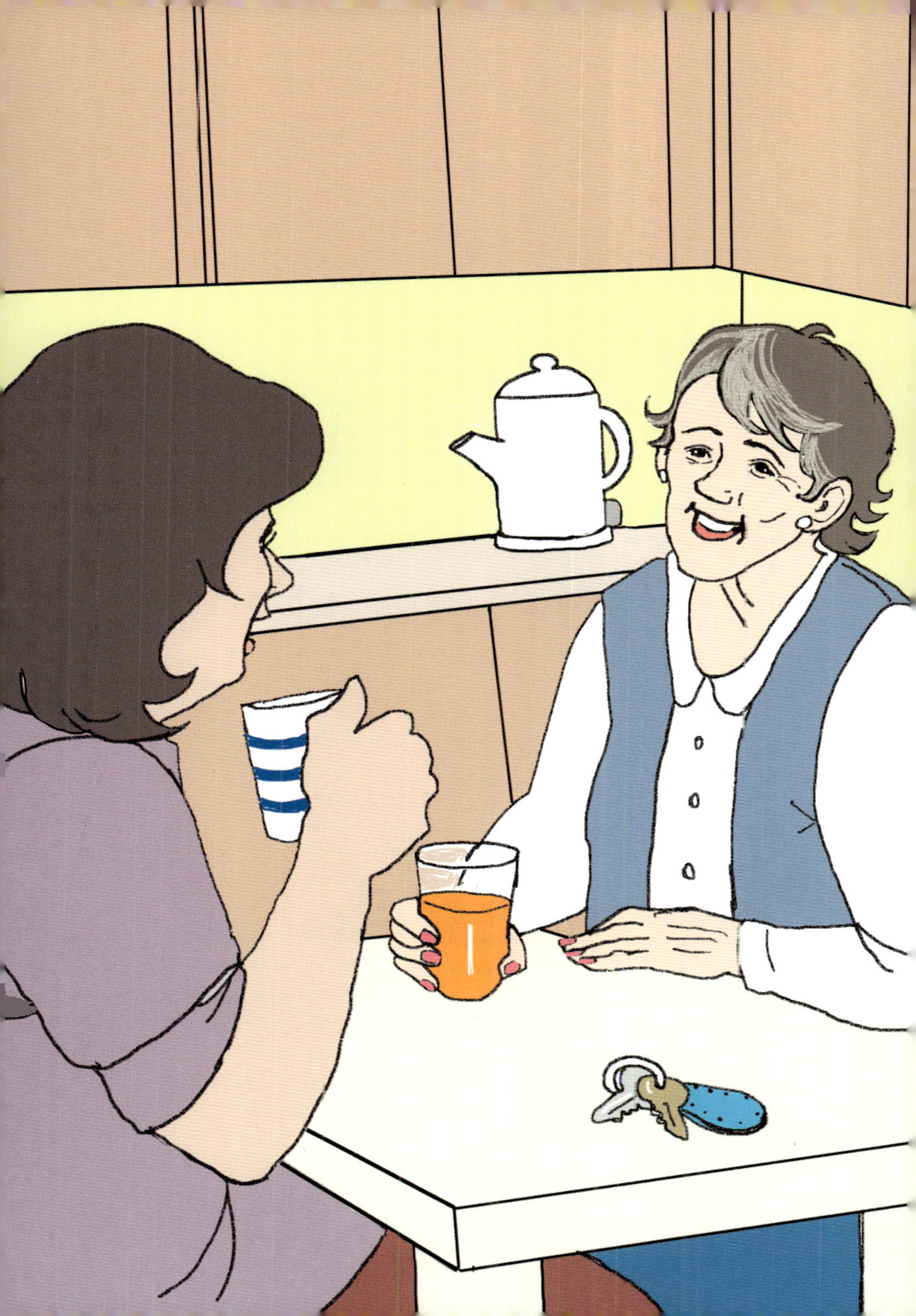

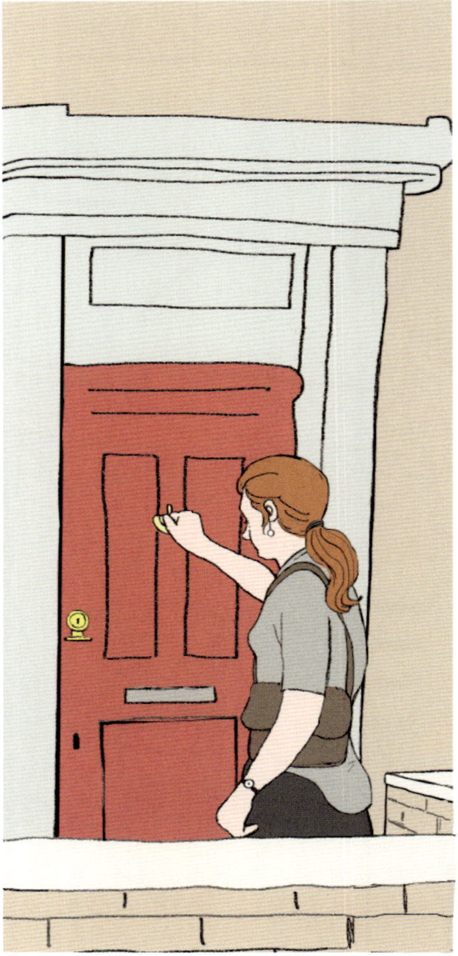

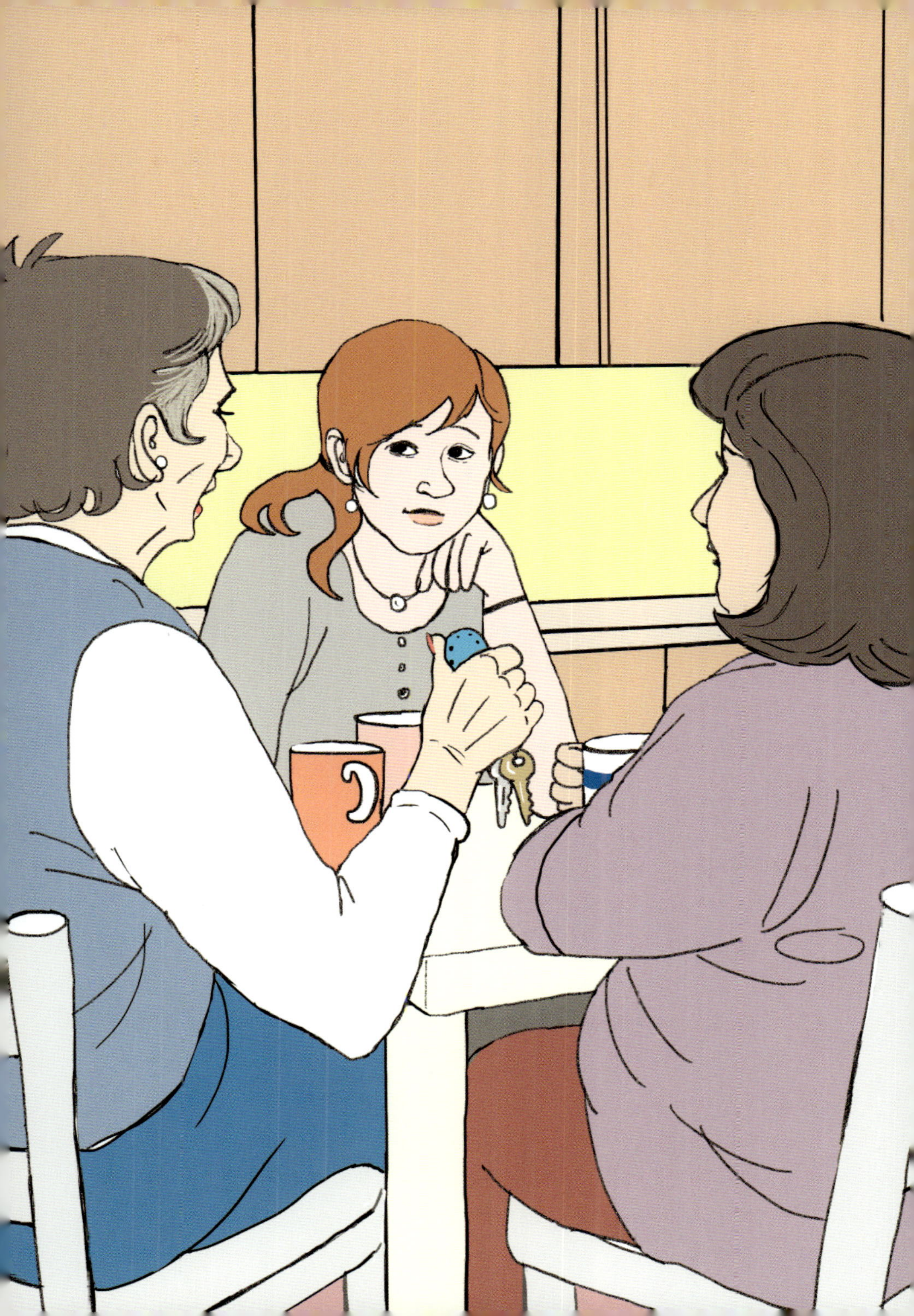

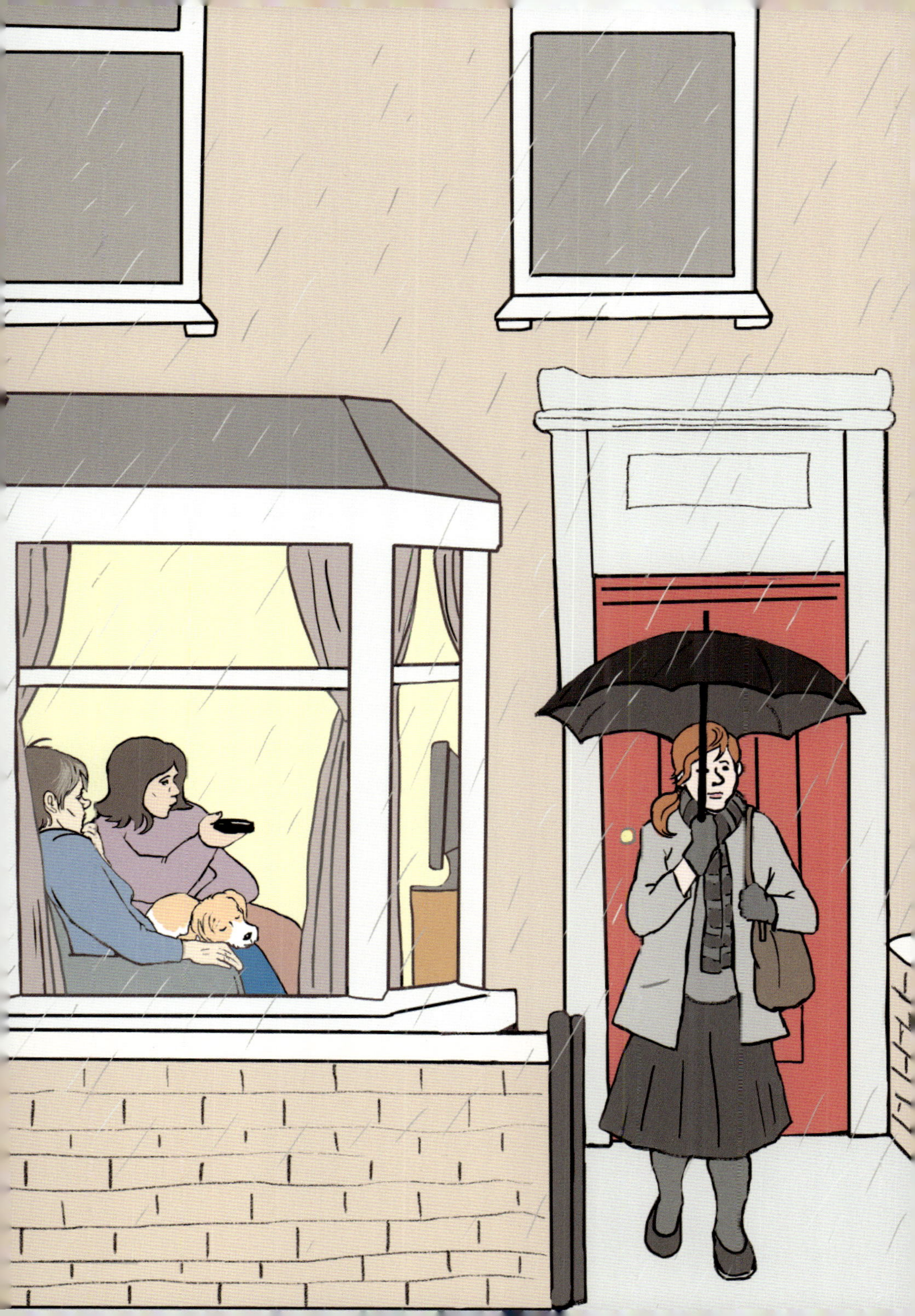

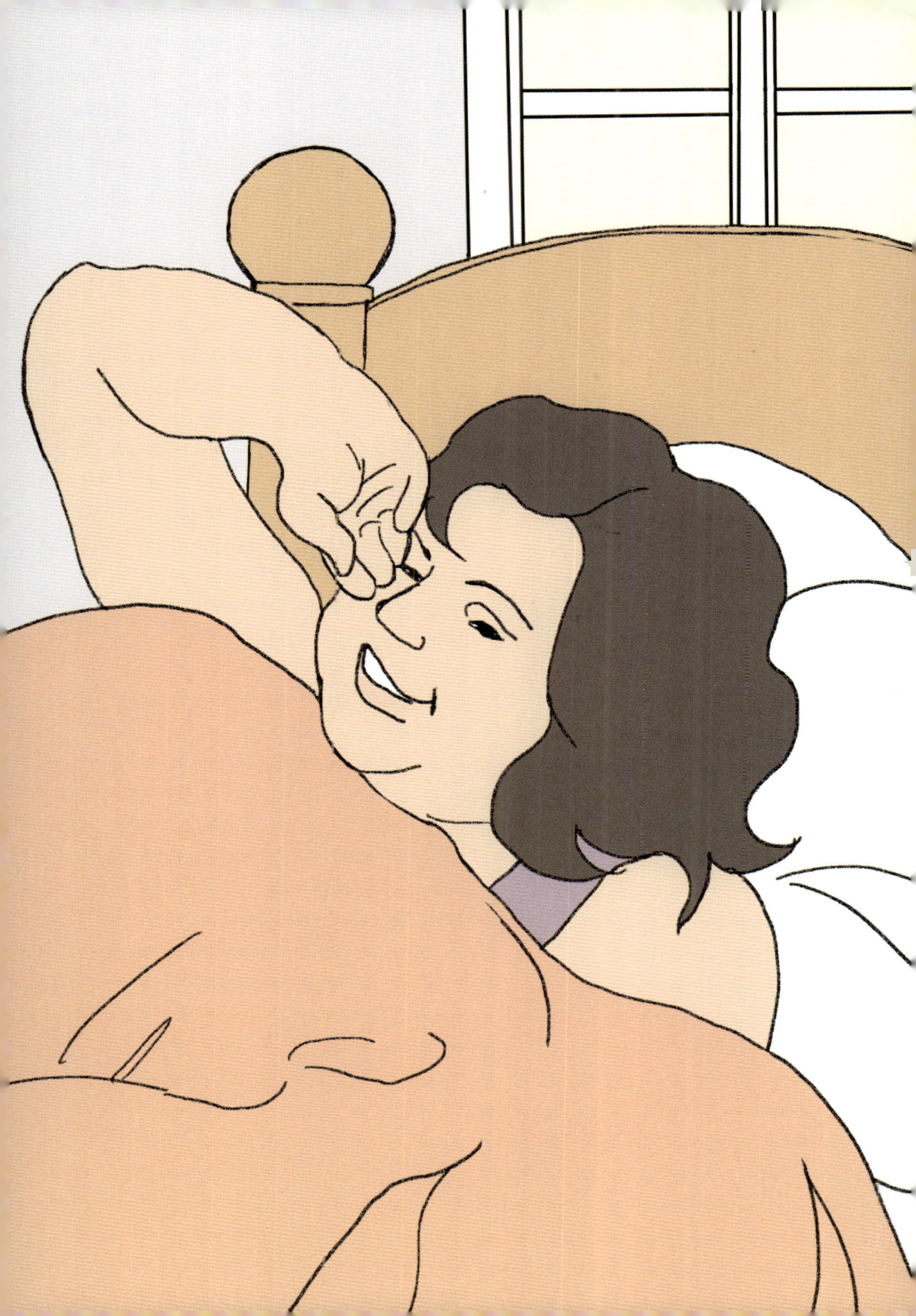

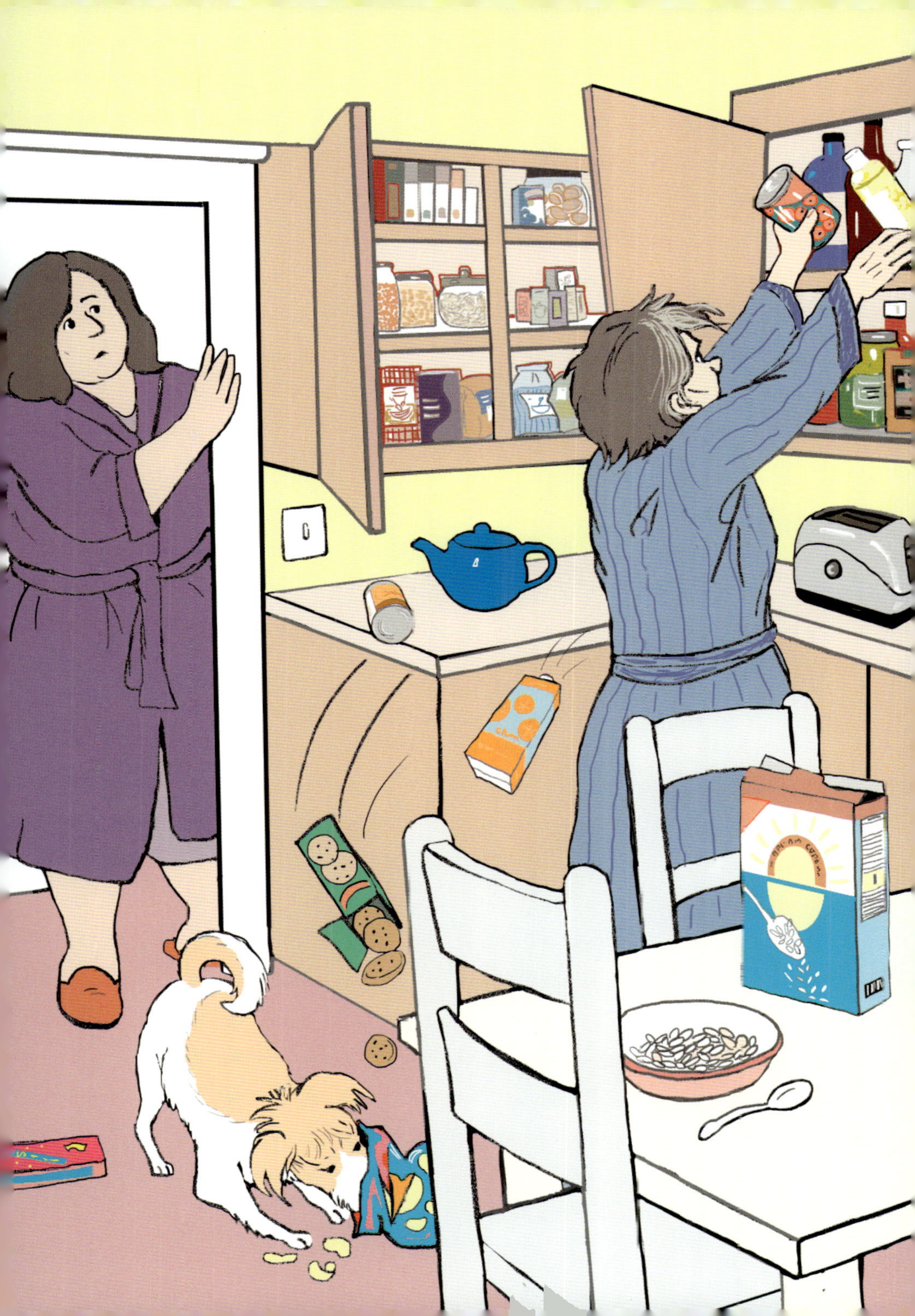

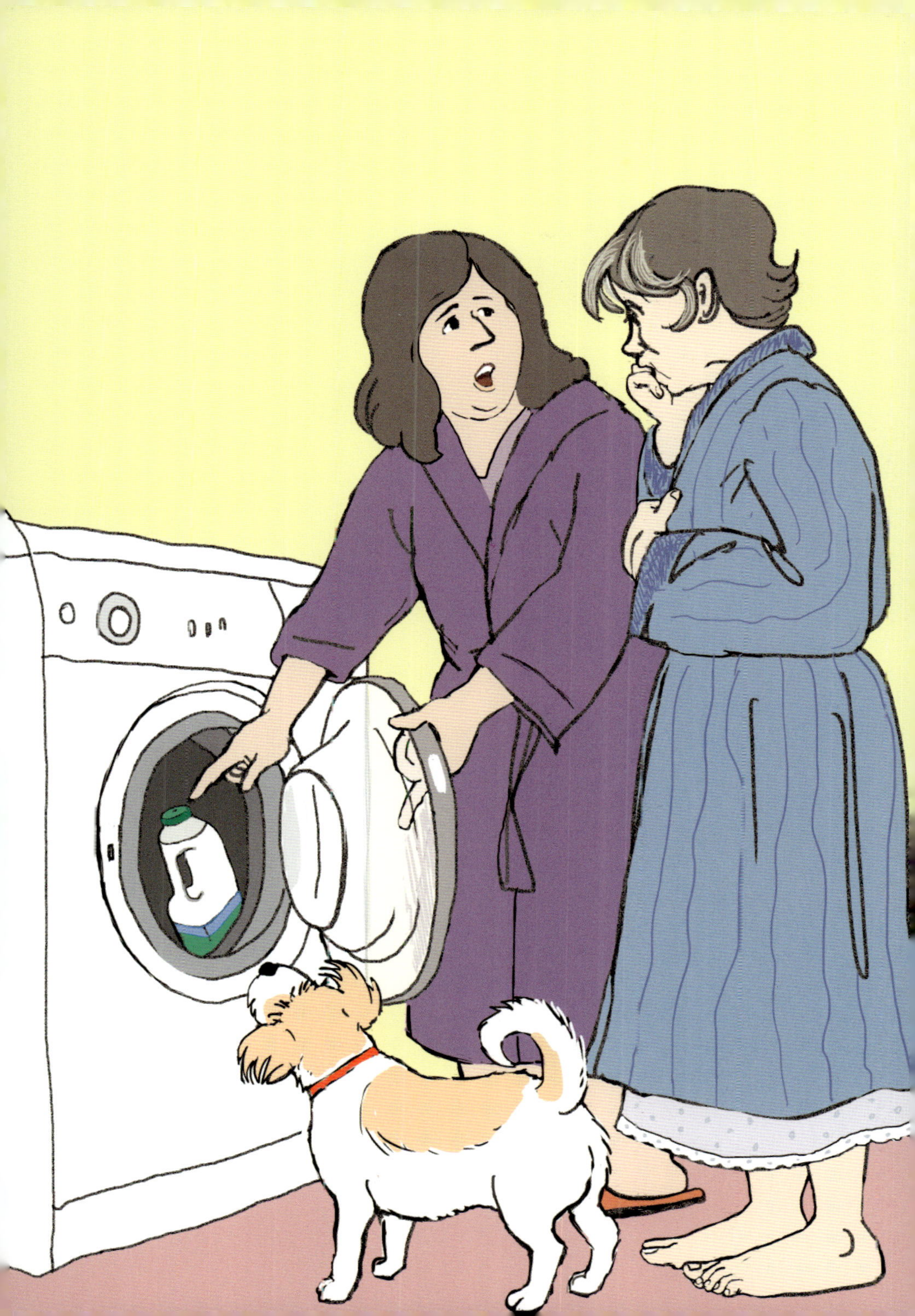

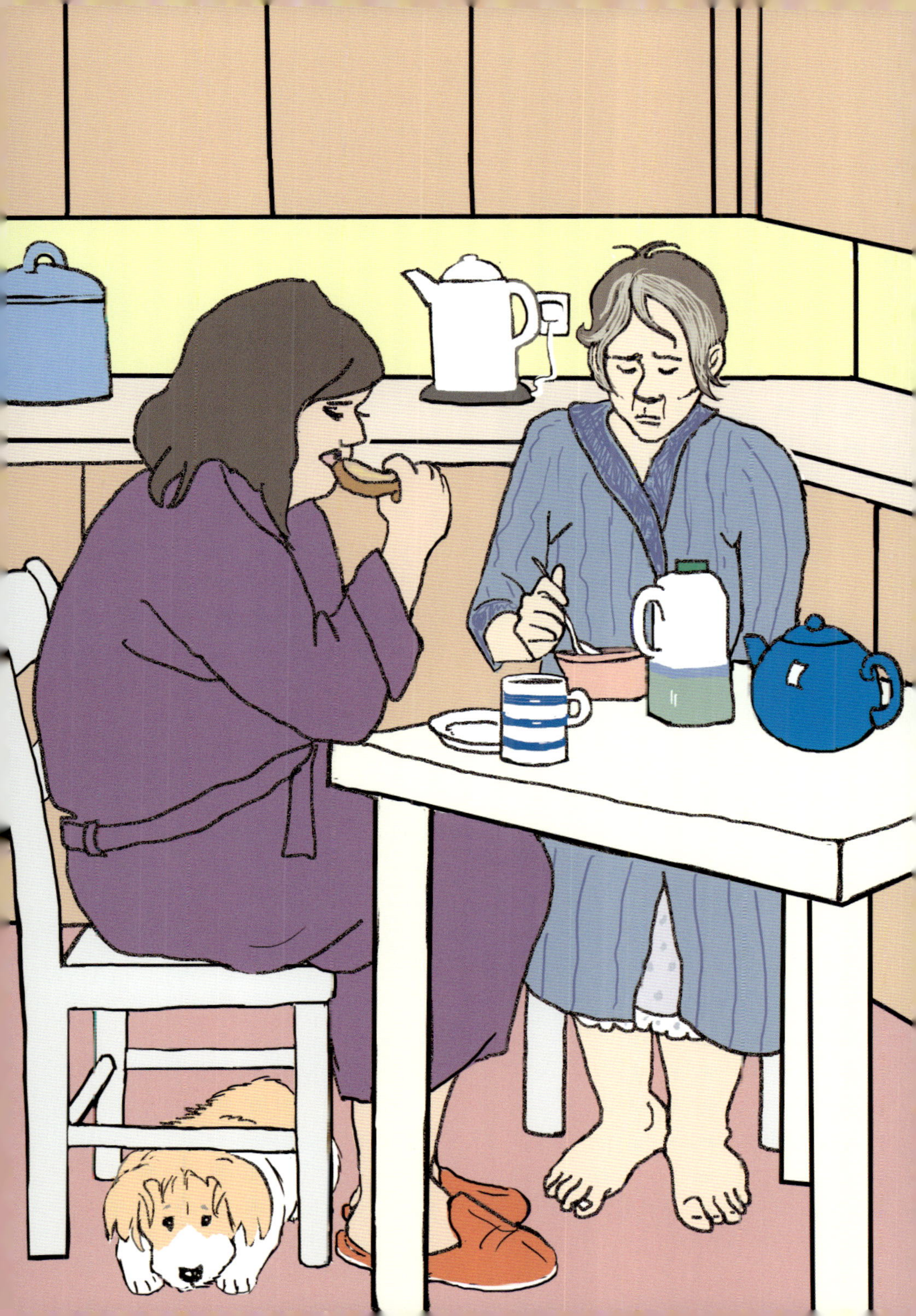

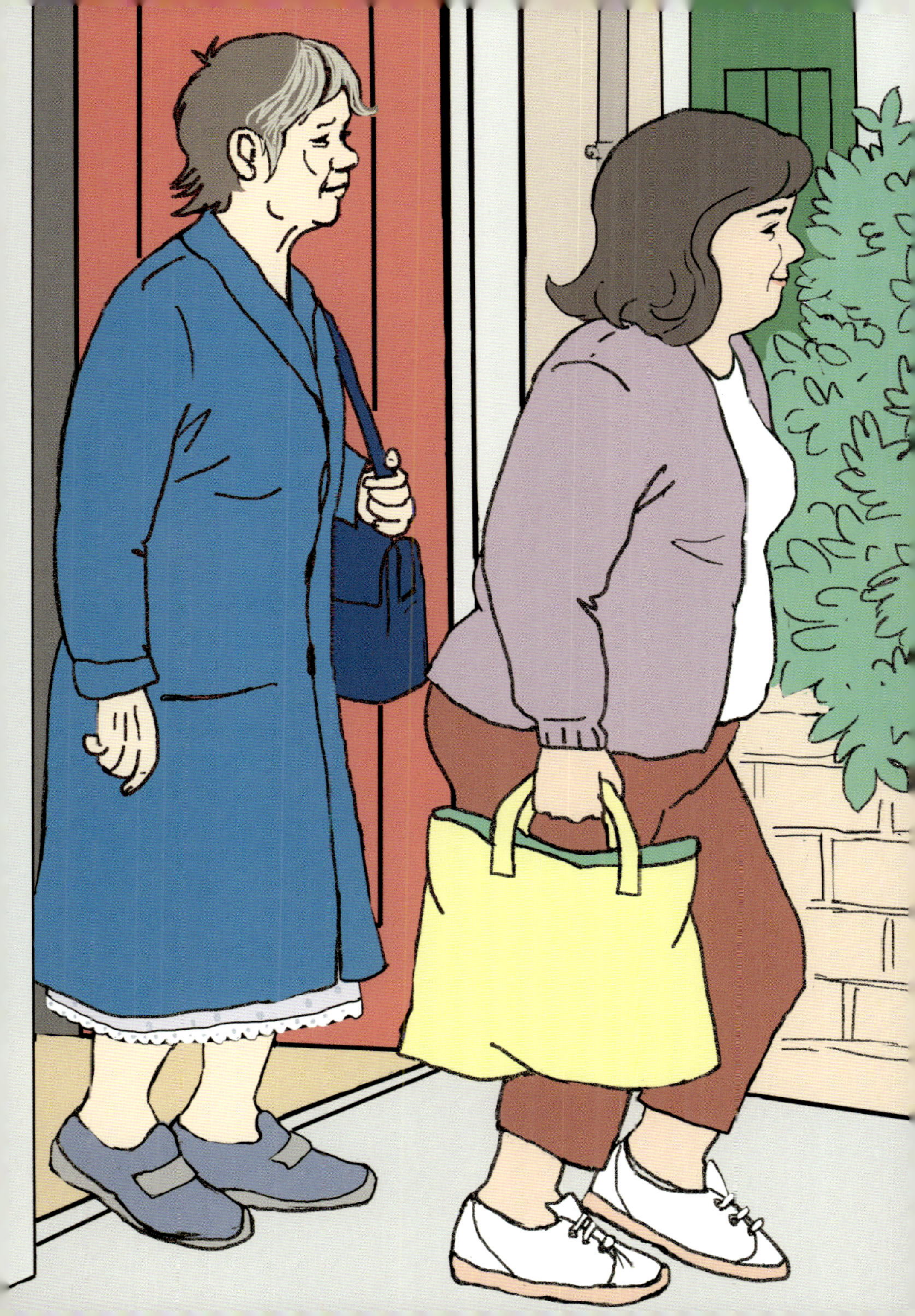

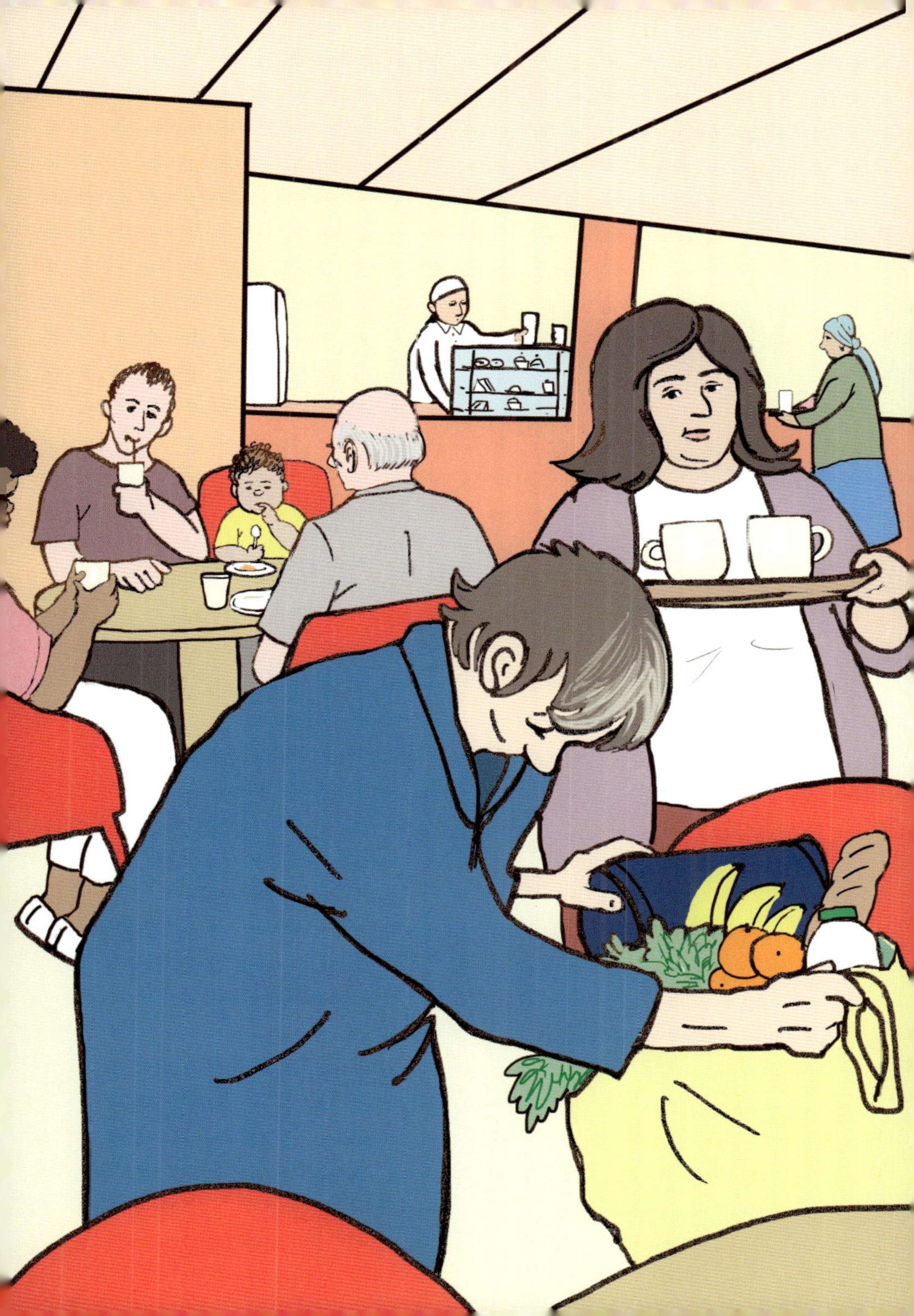

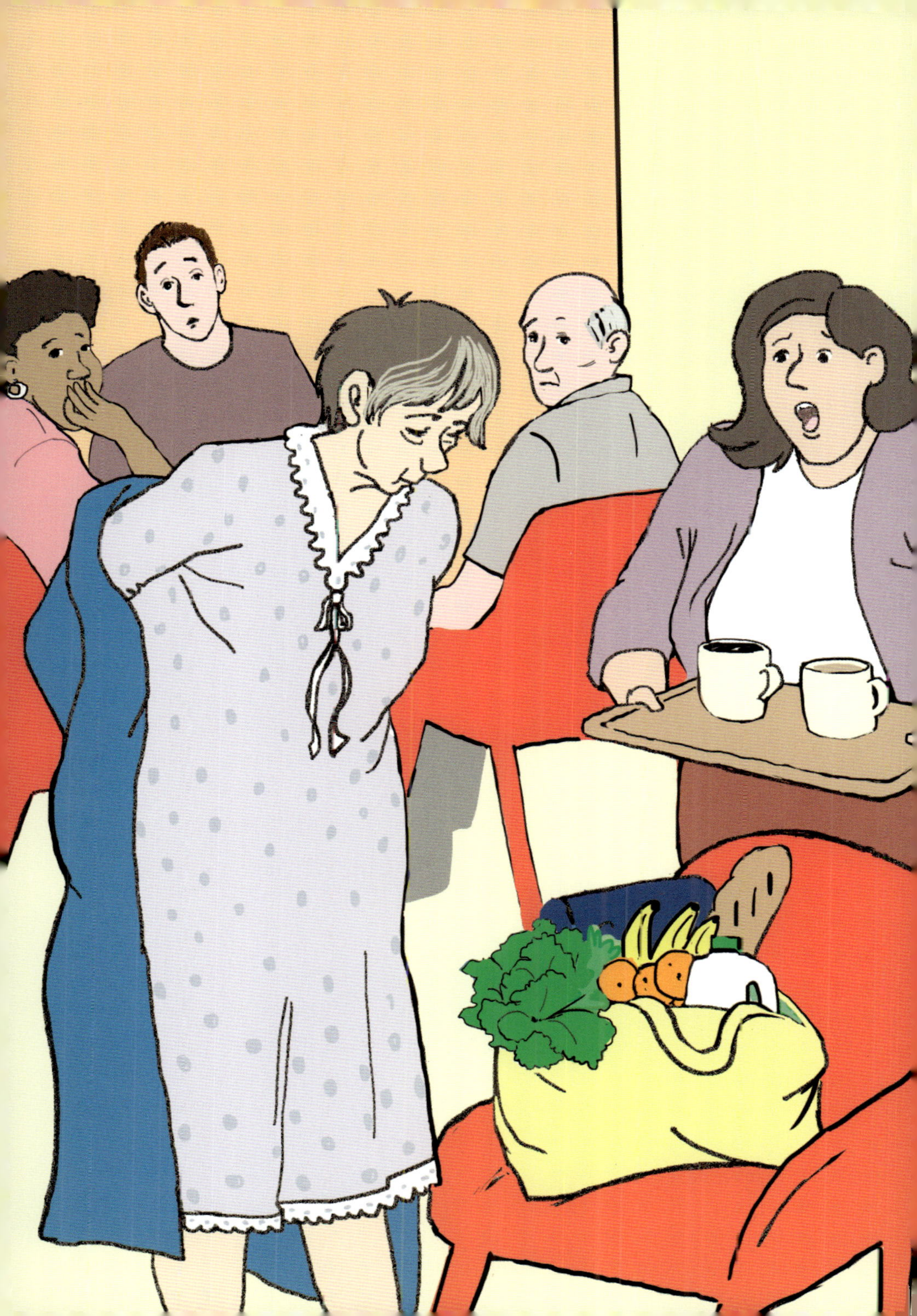

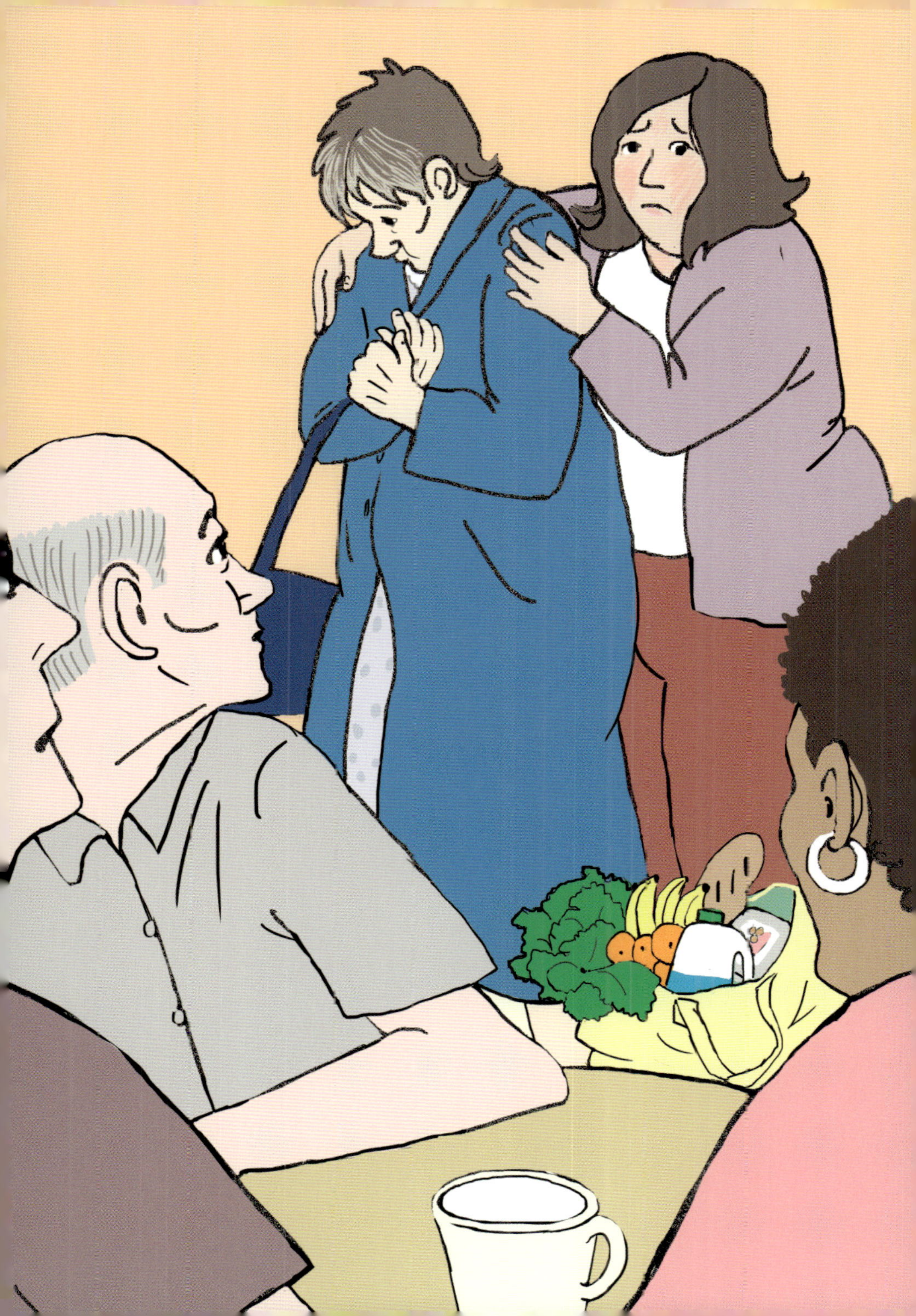

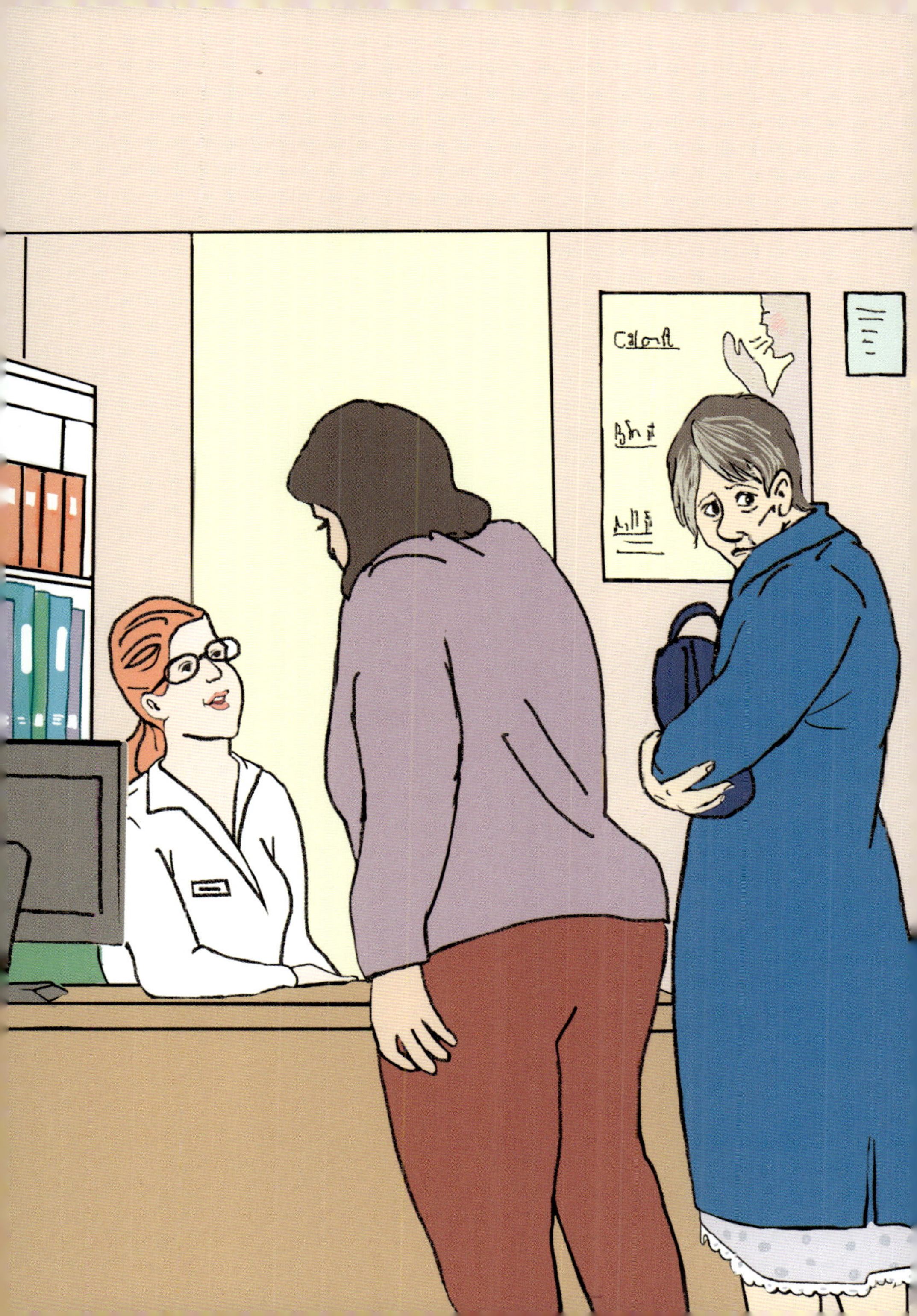

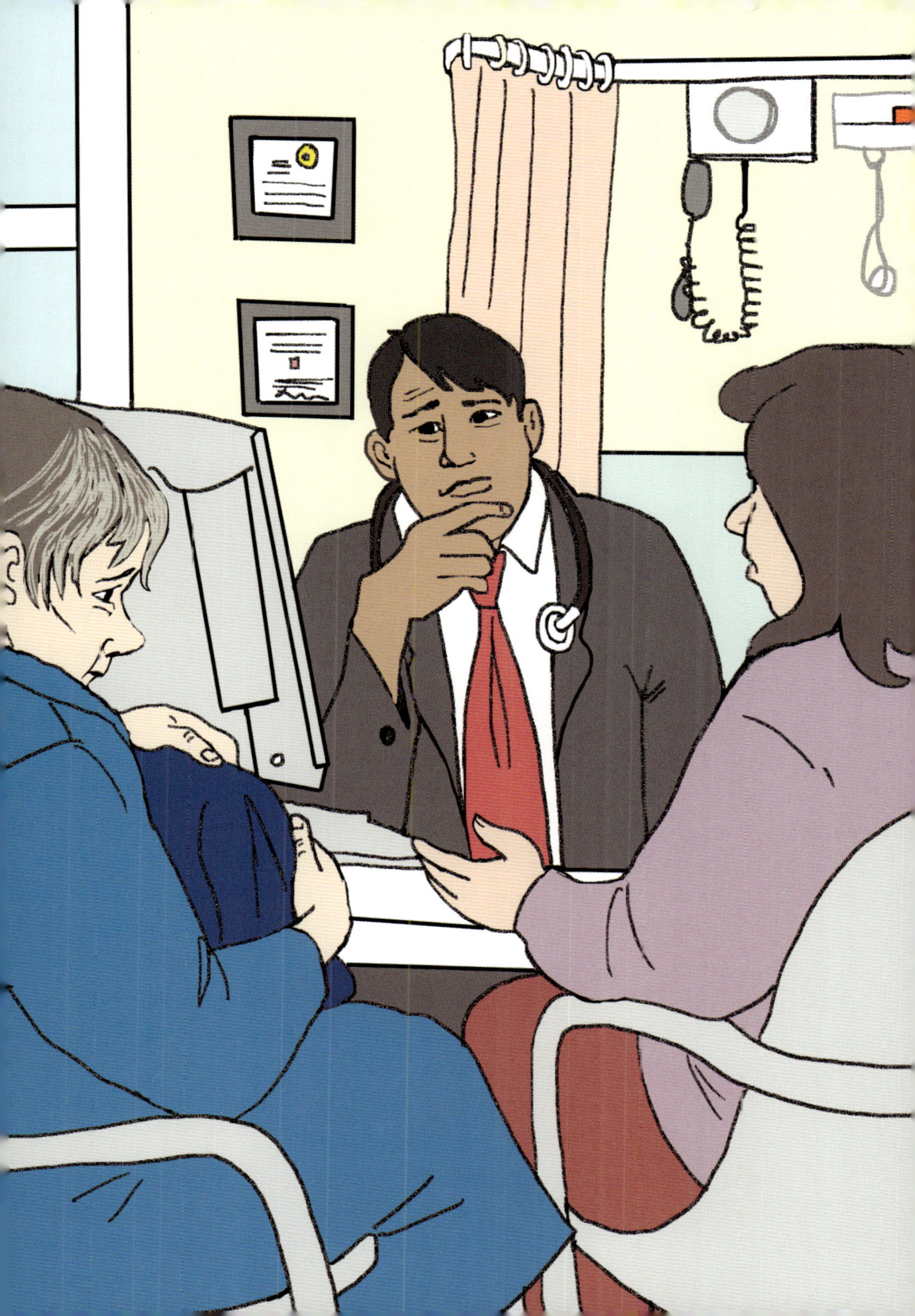

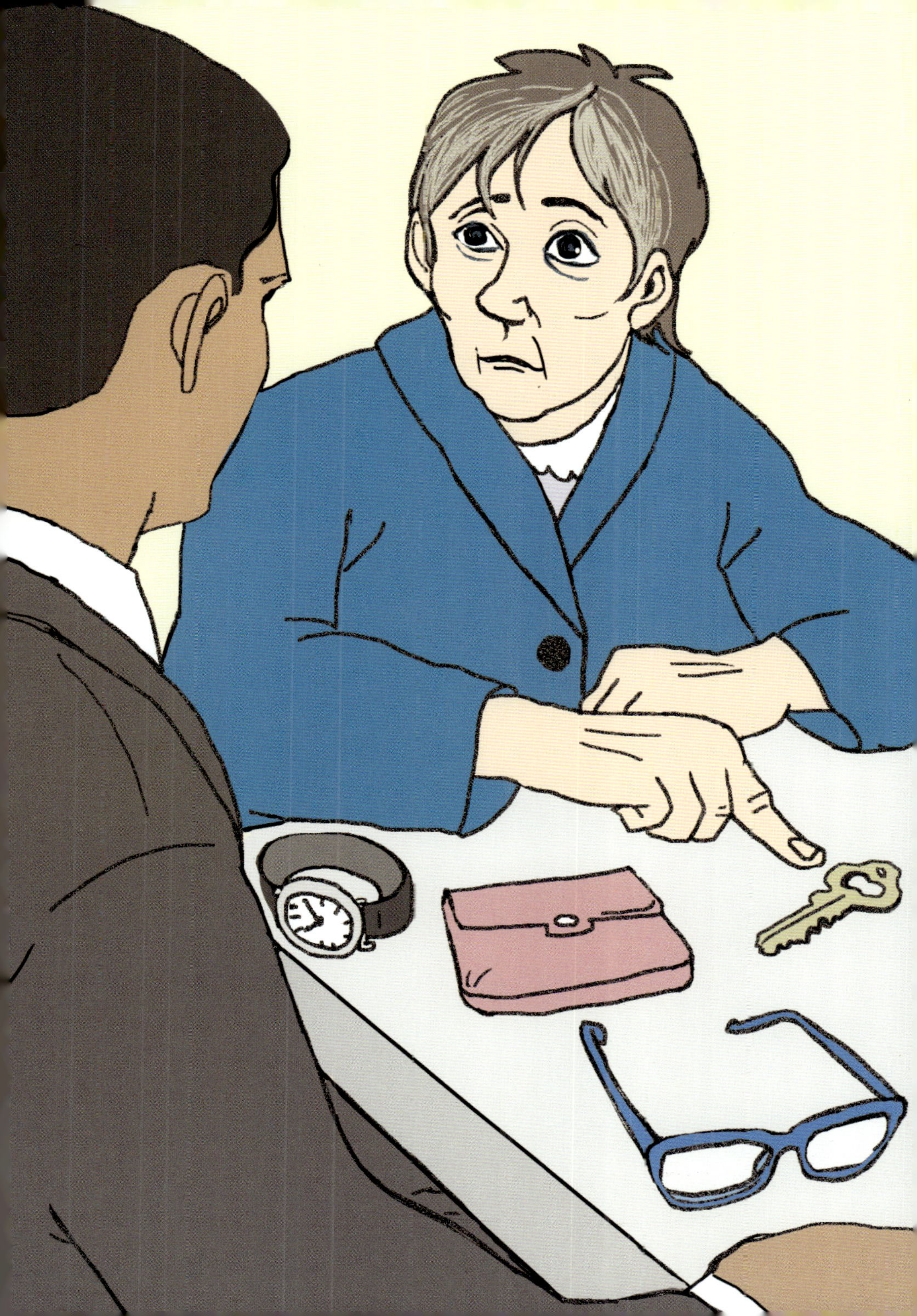

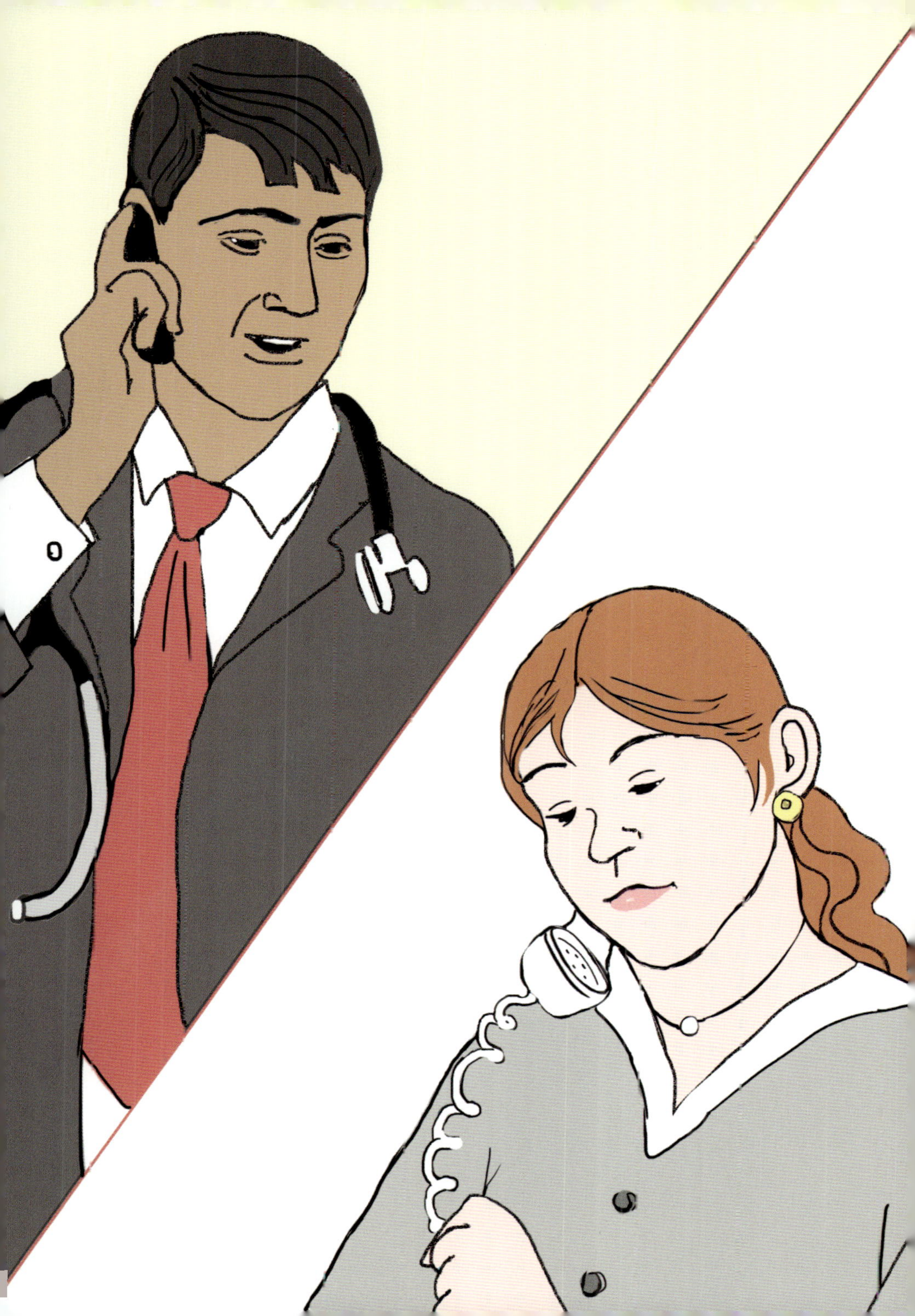

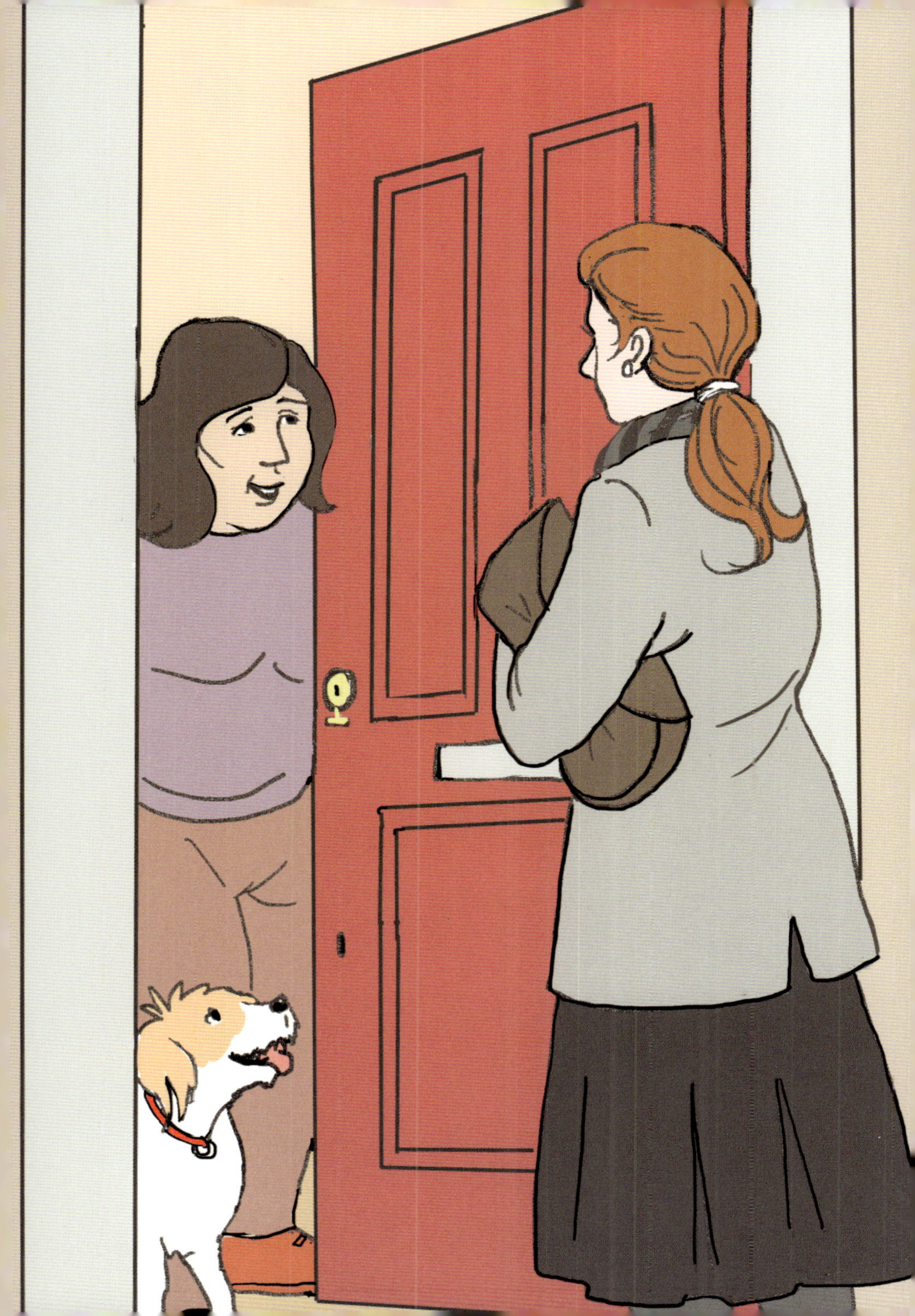

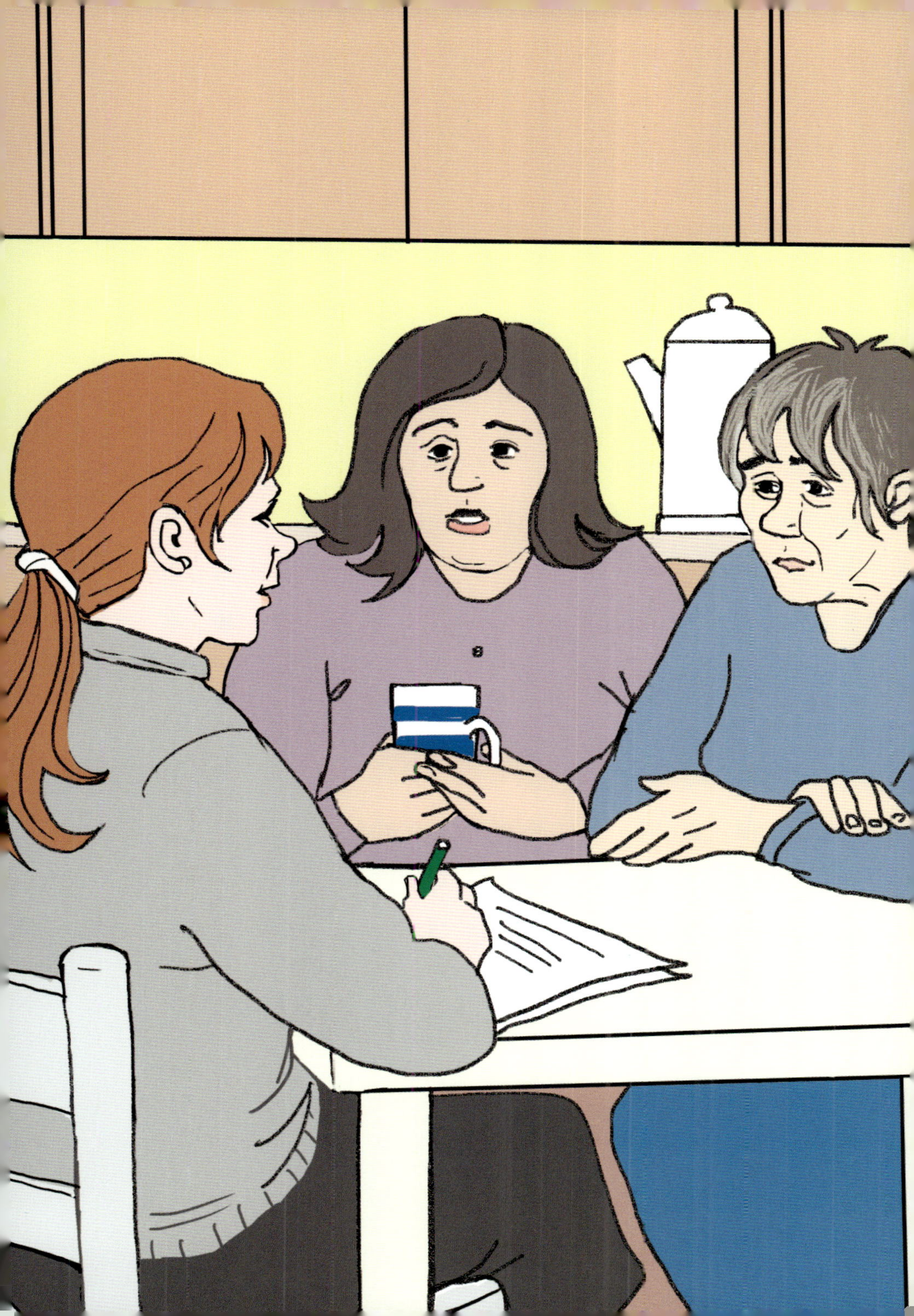

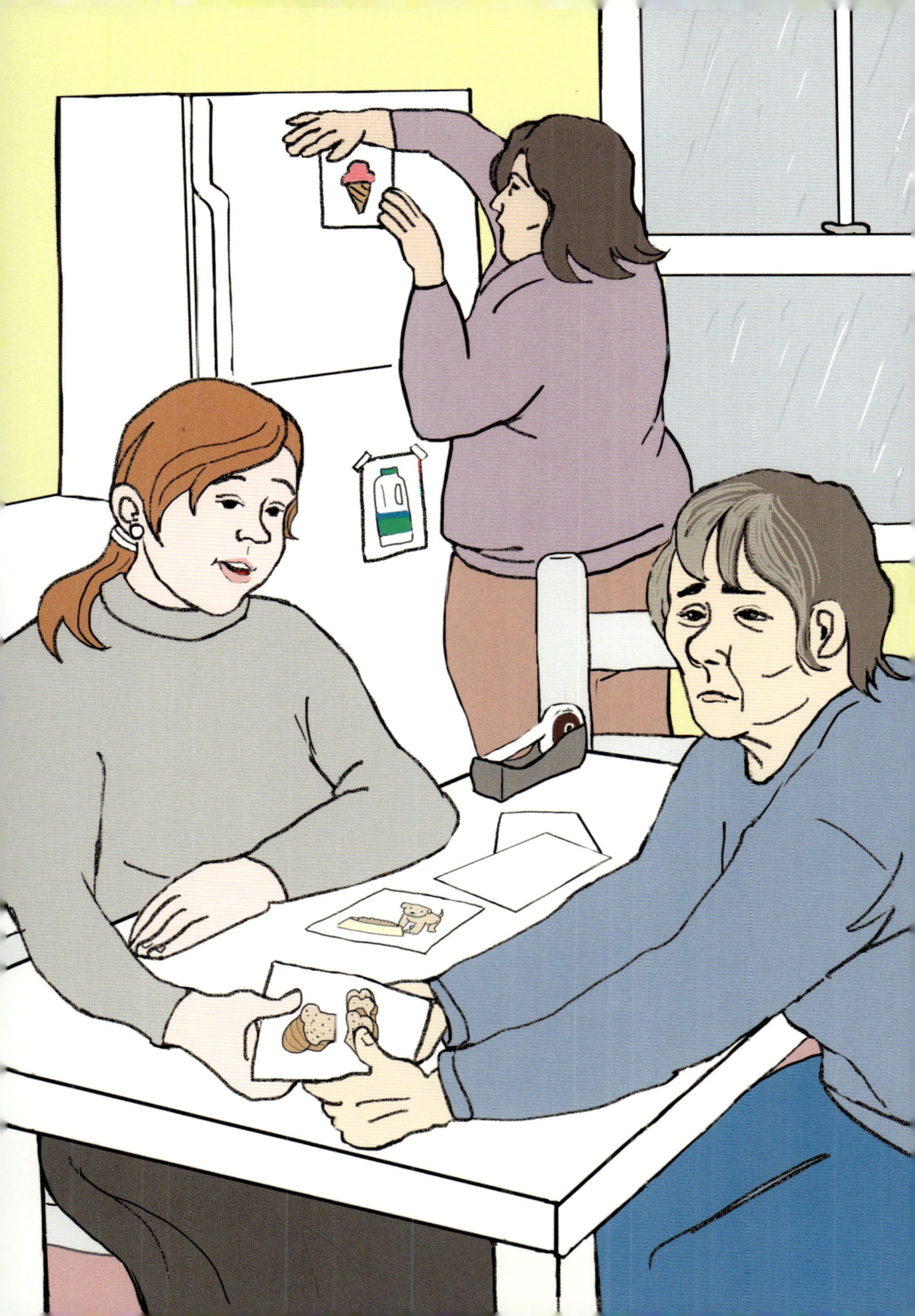

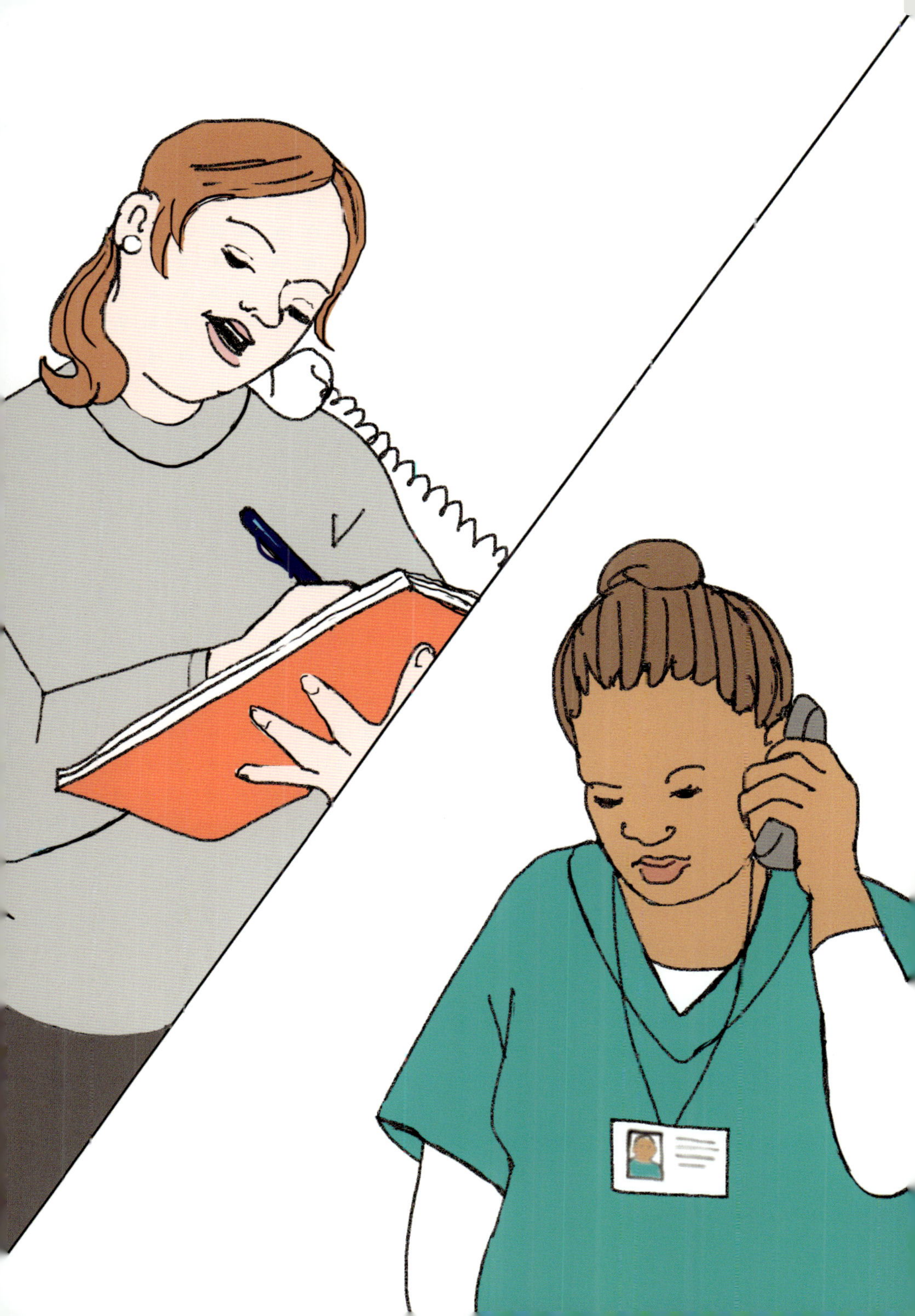

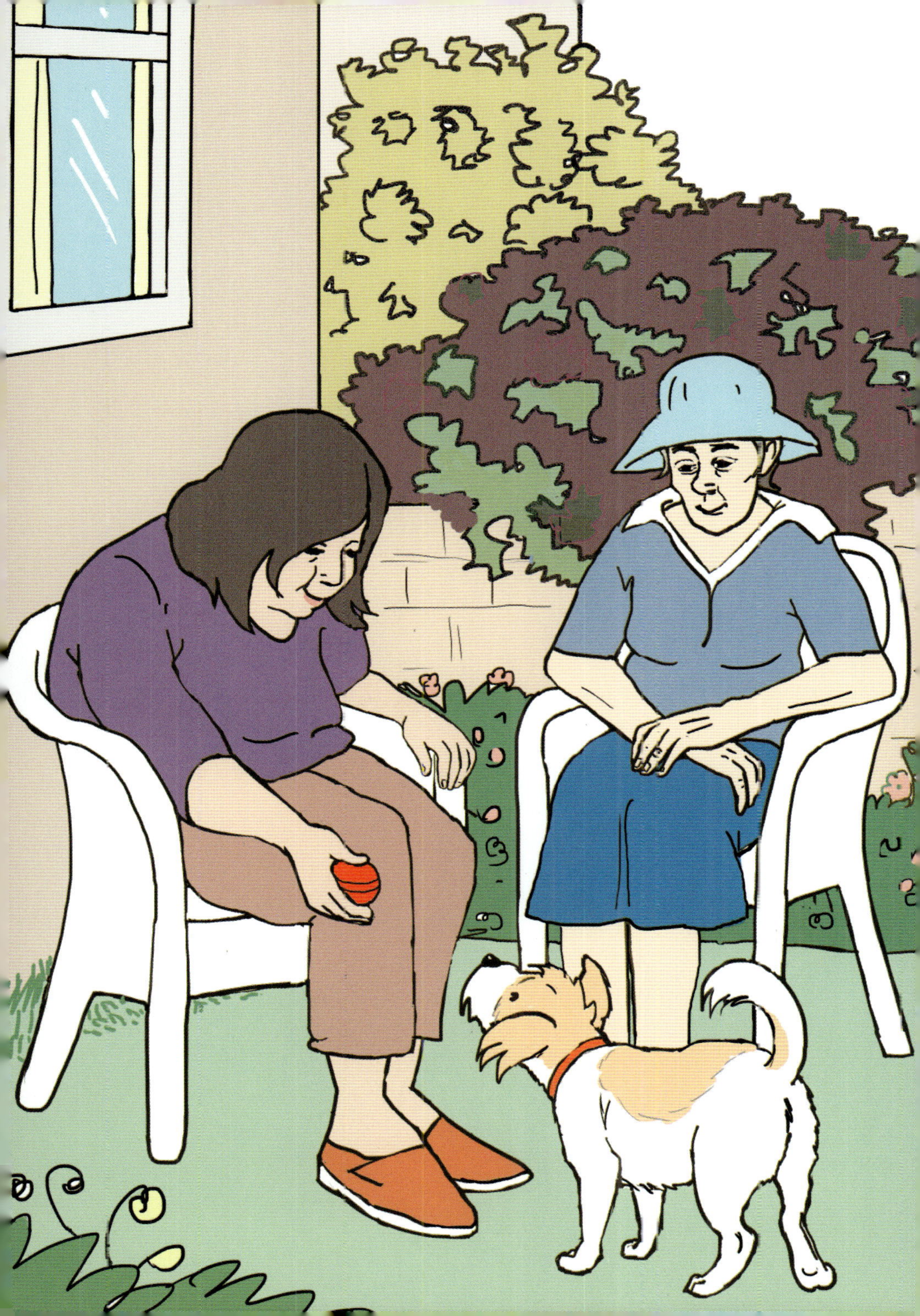

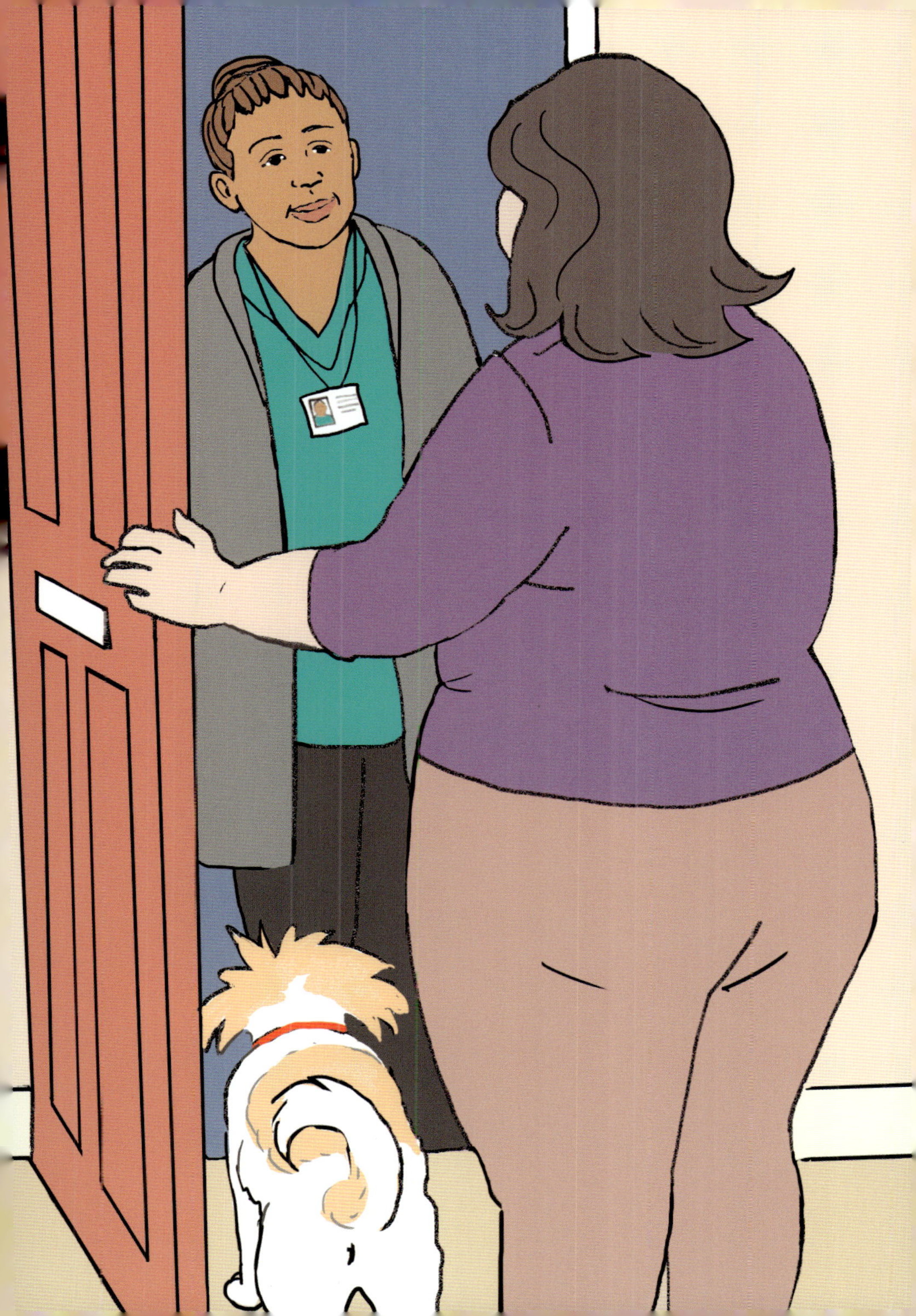

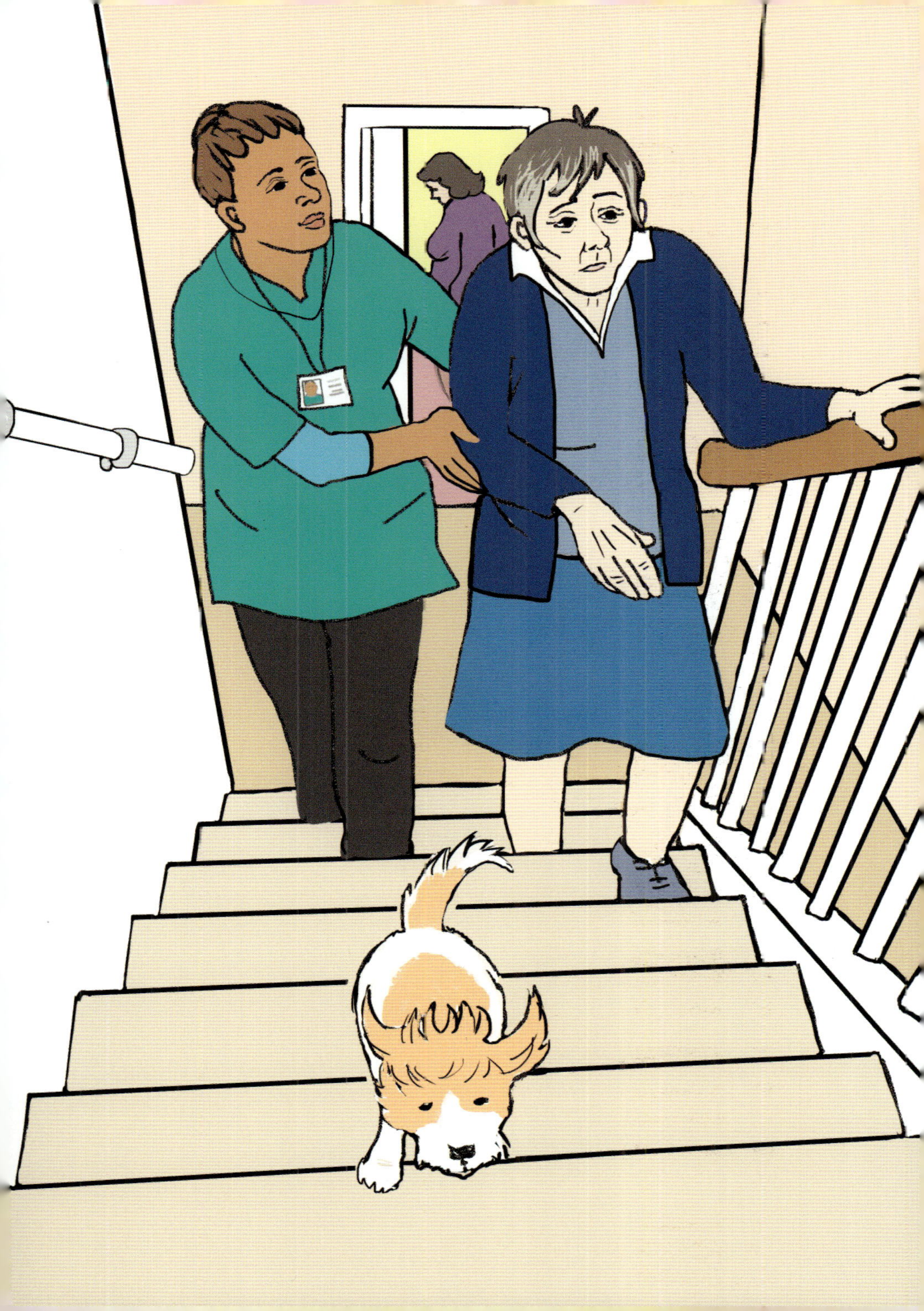

27

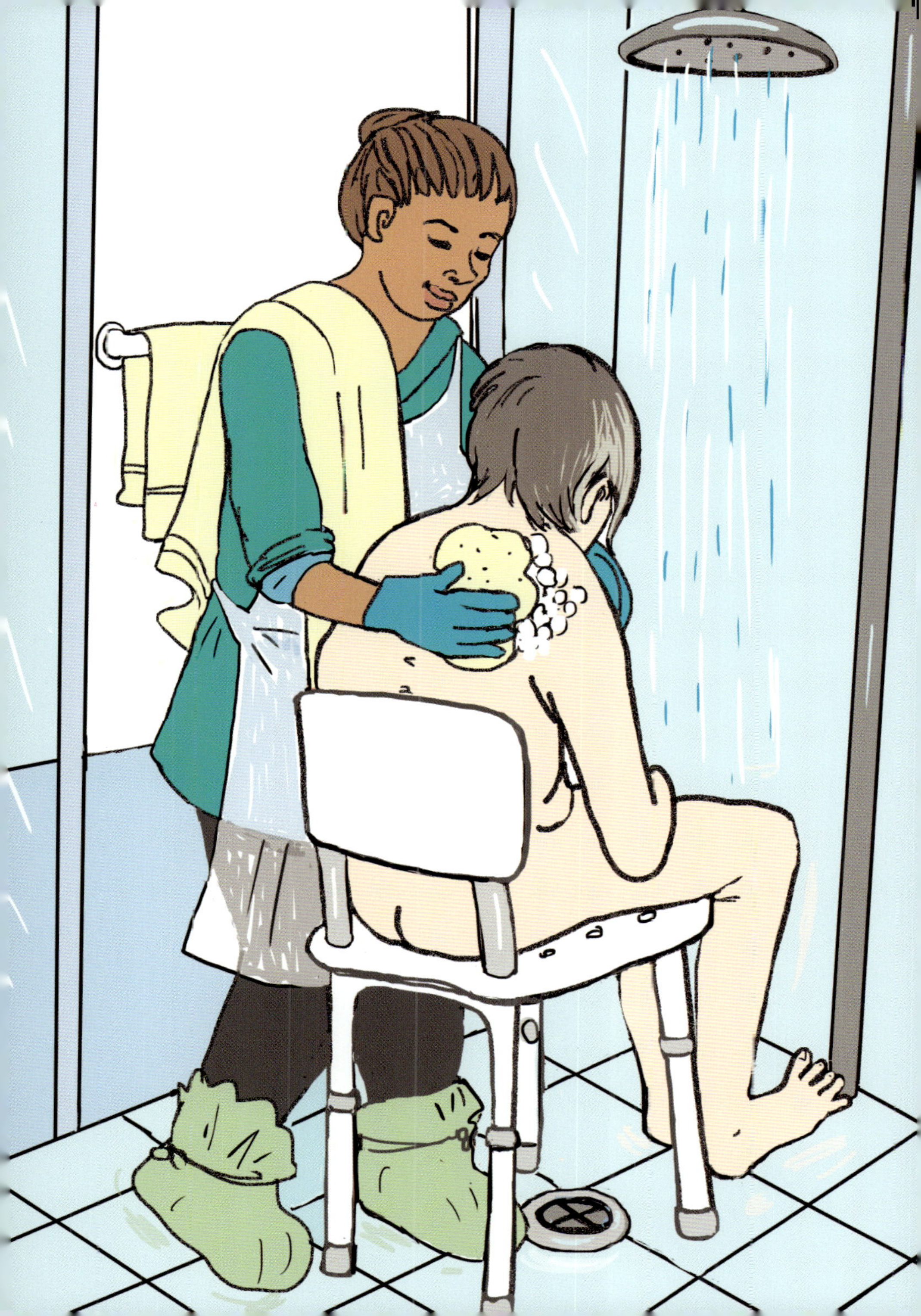

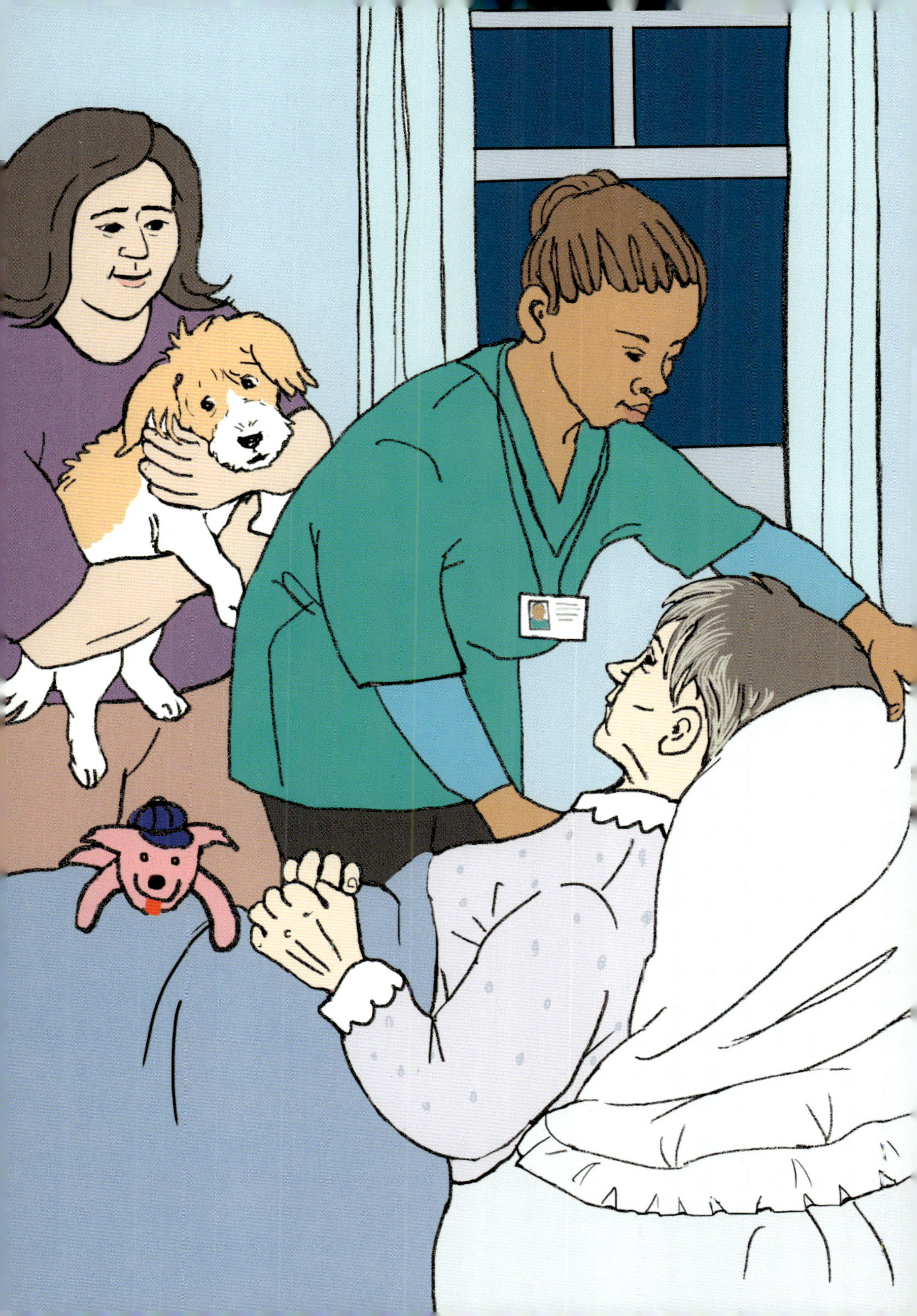

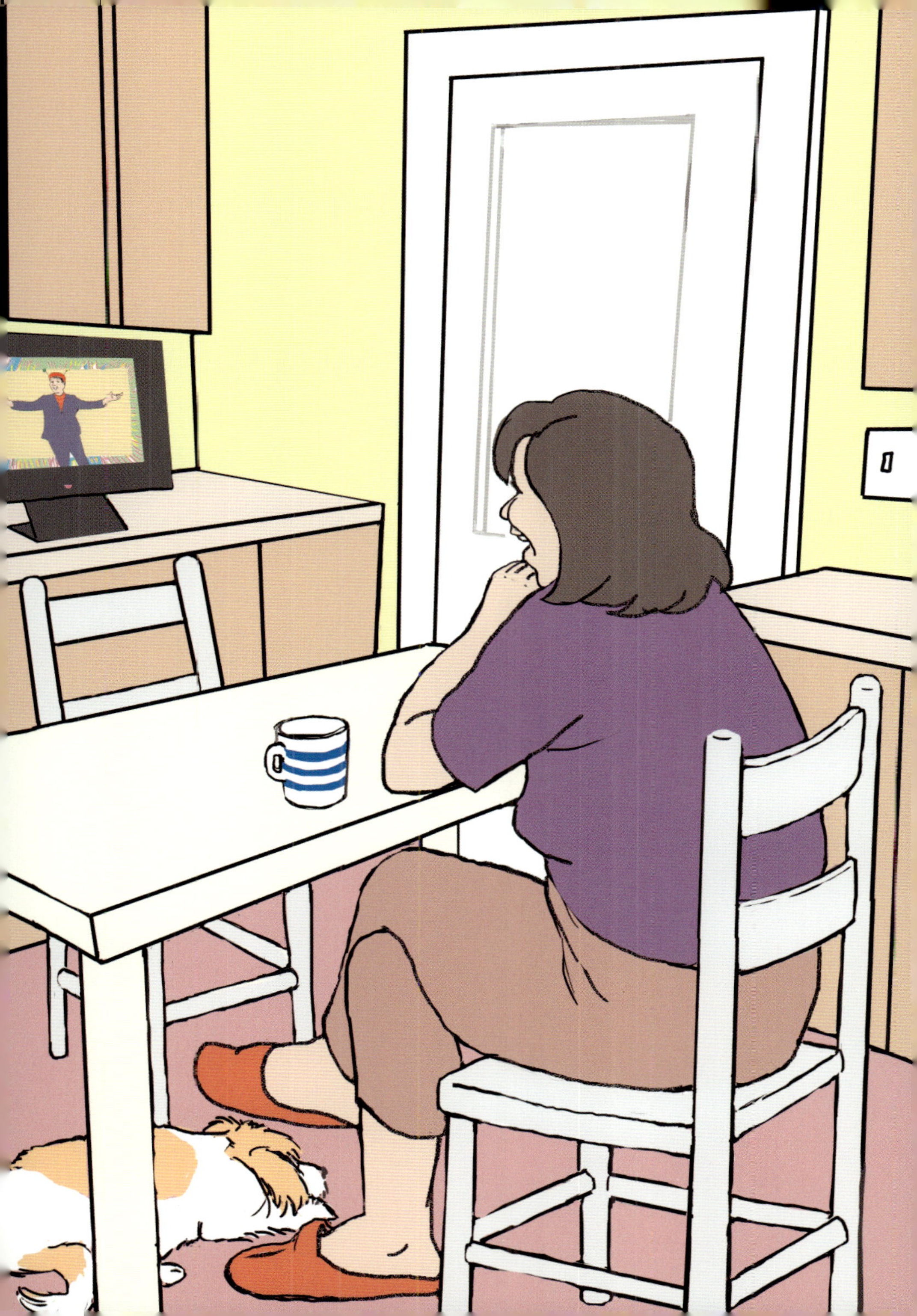

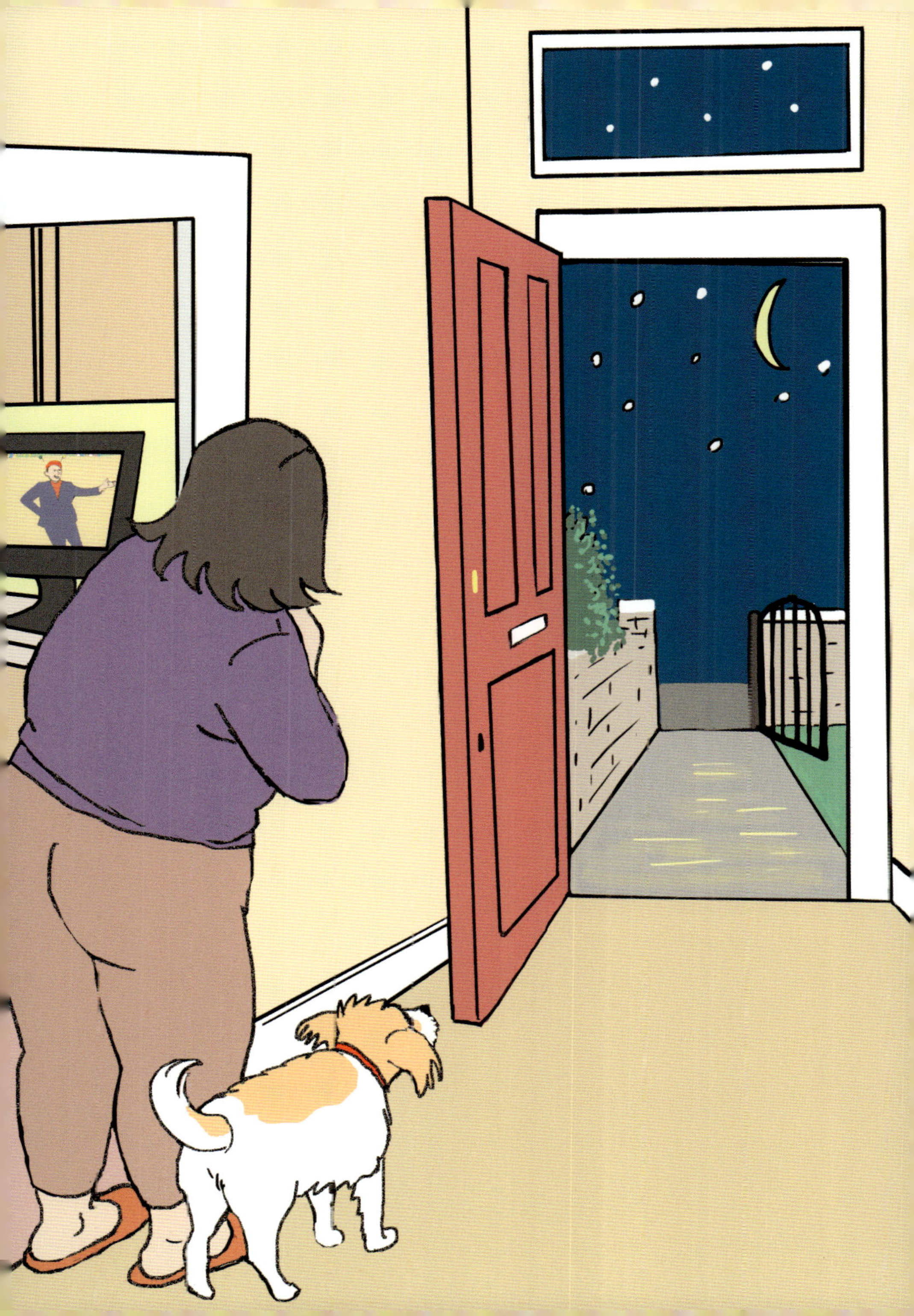

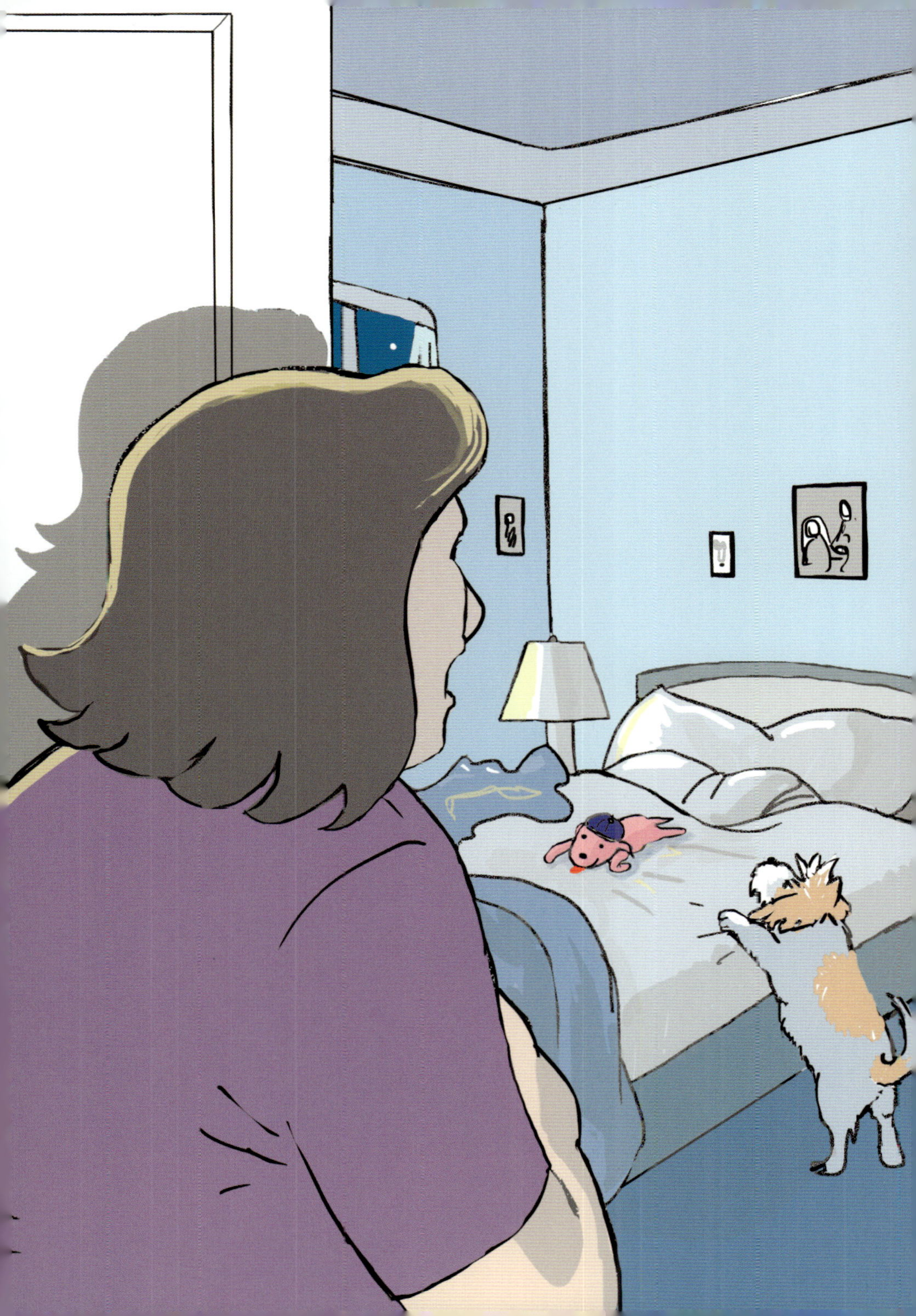

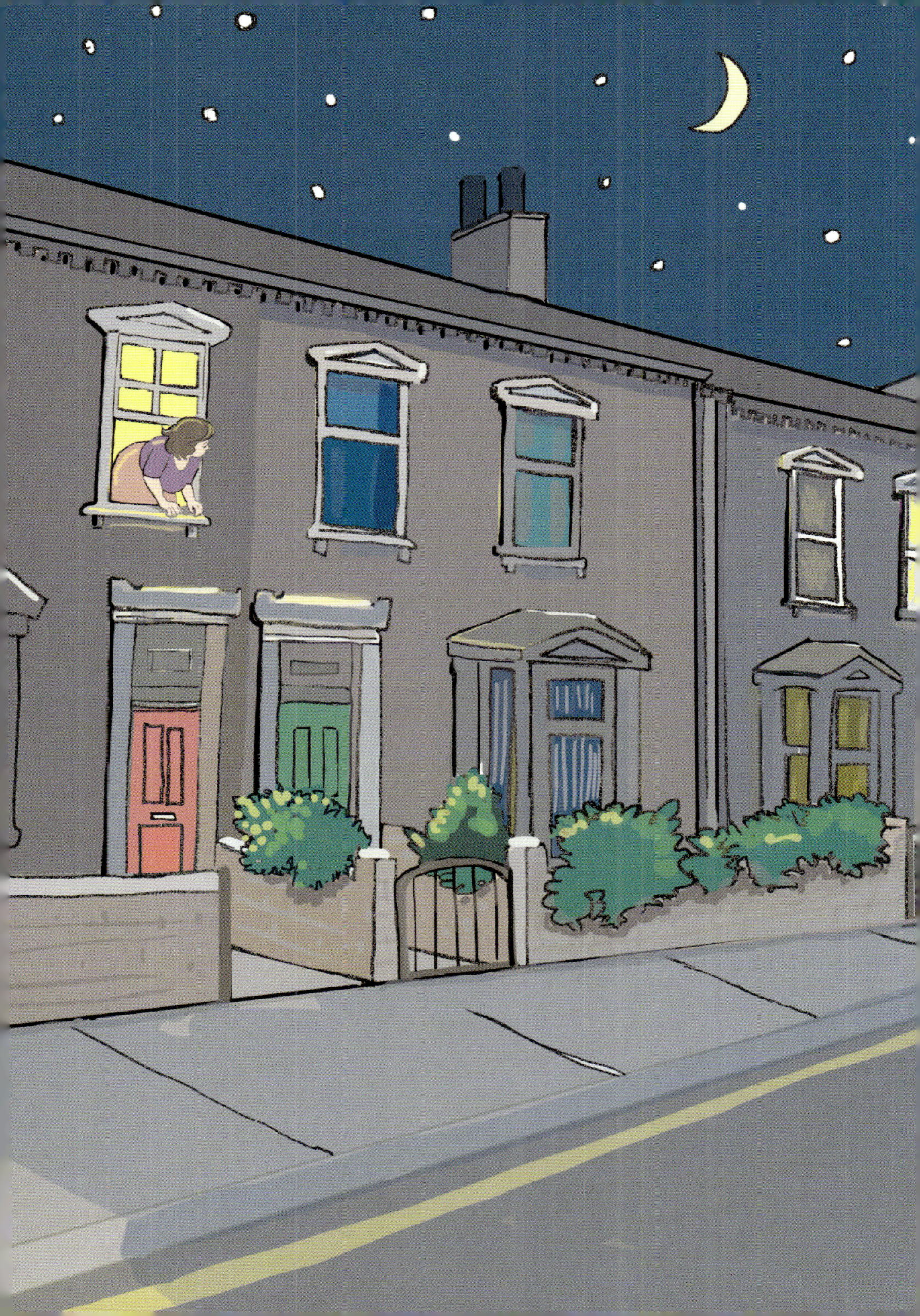

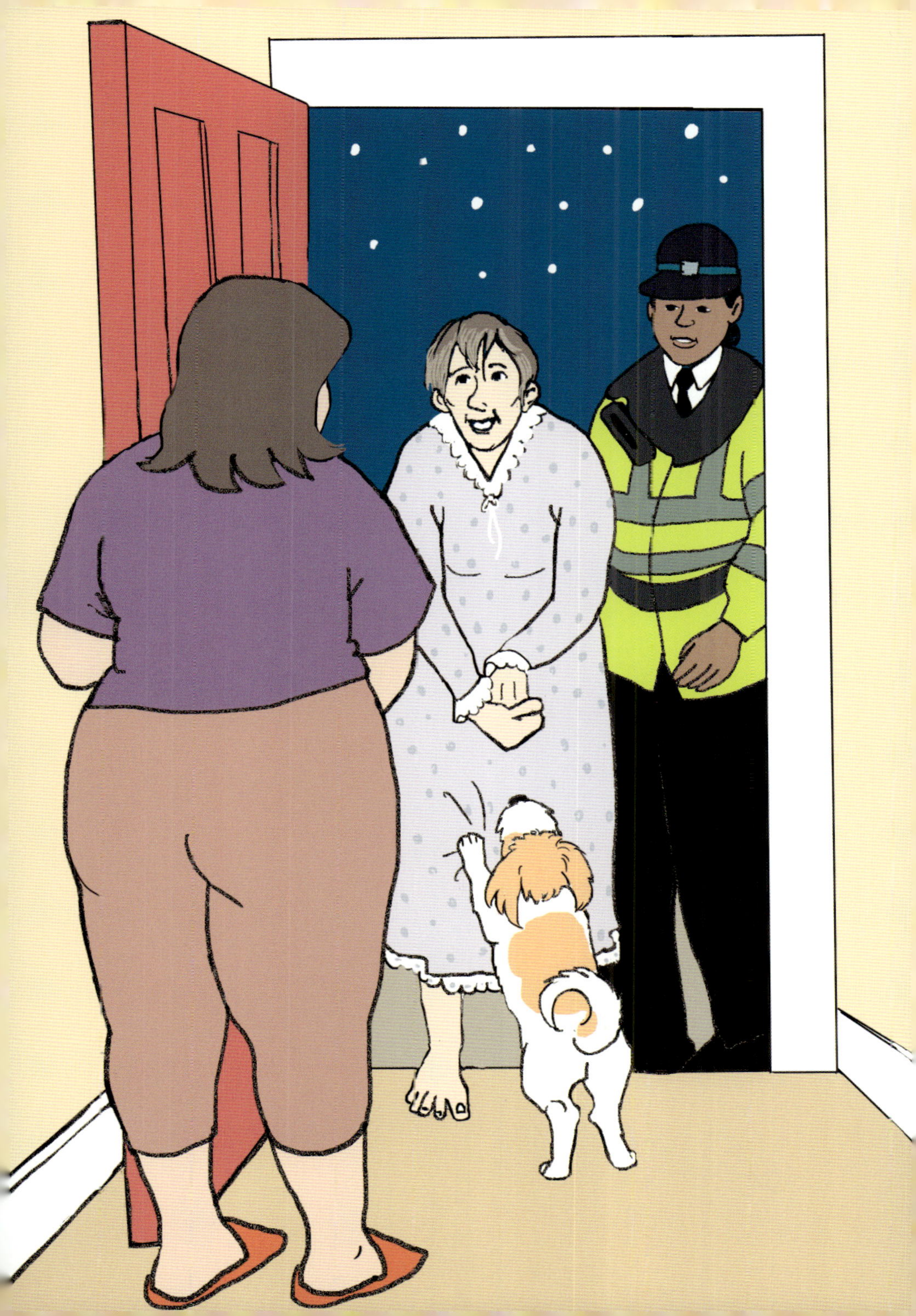

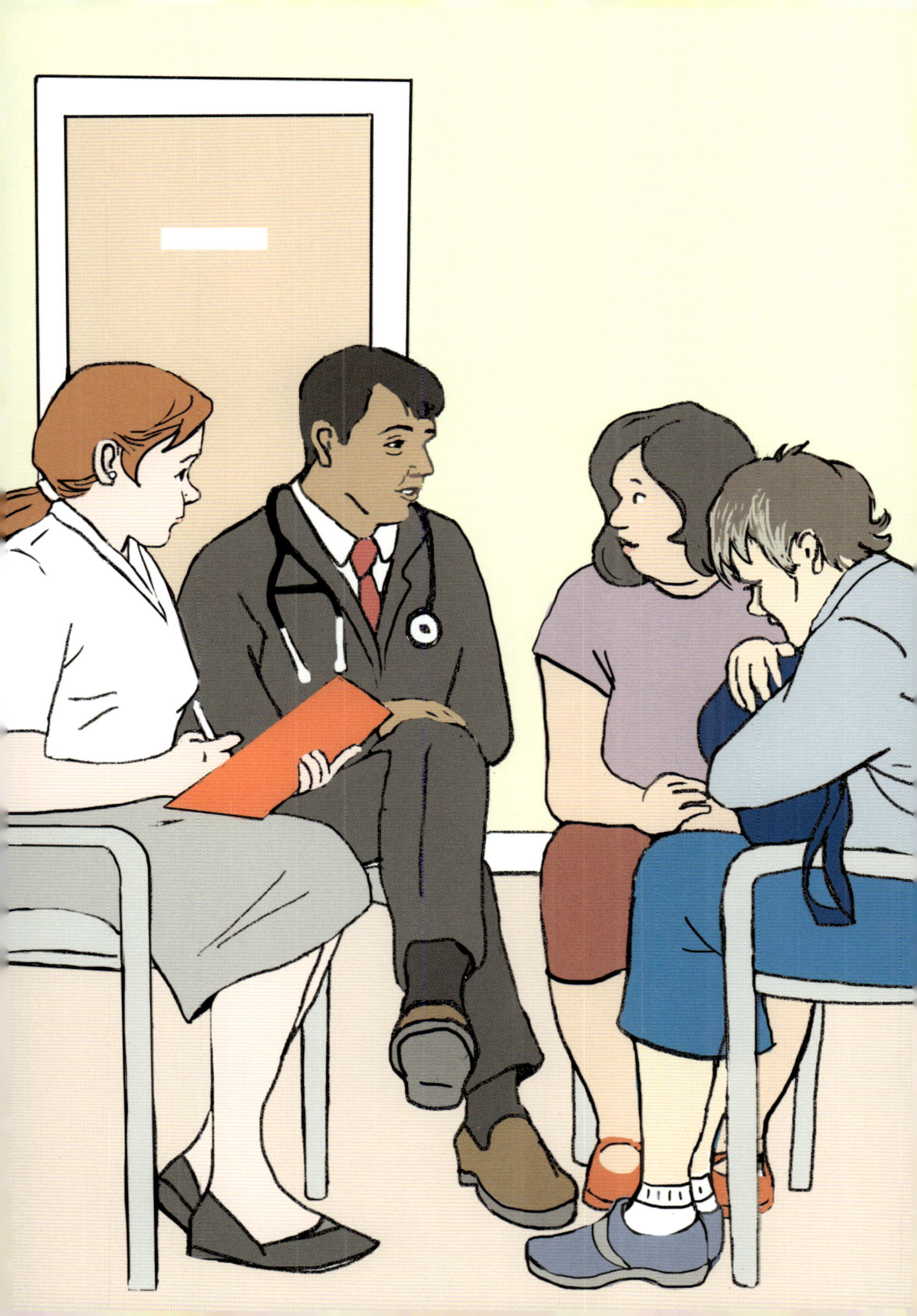

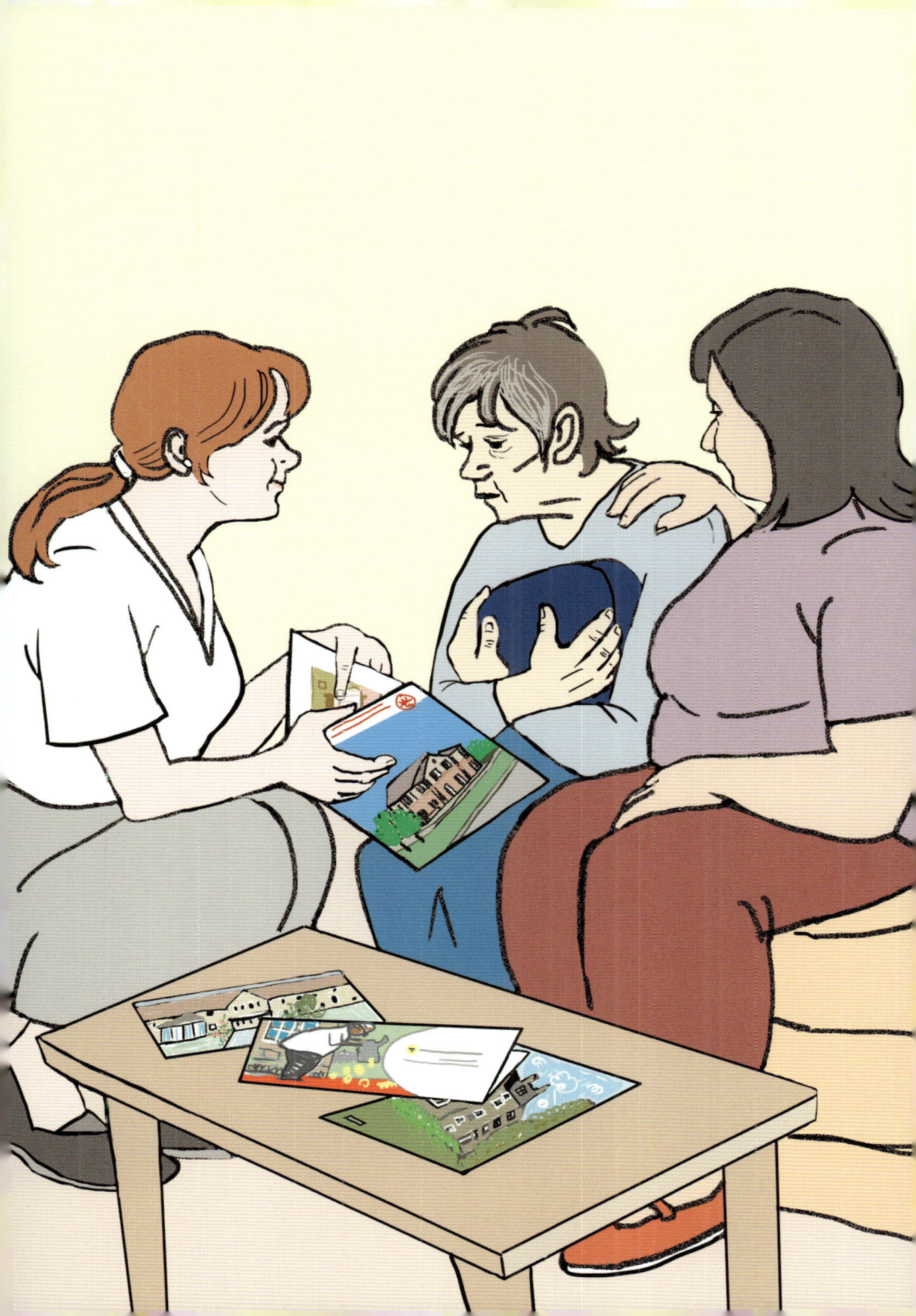

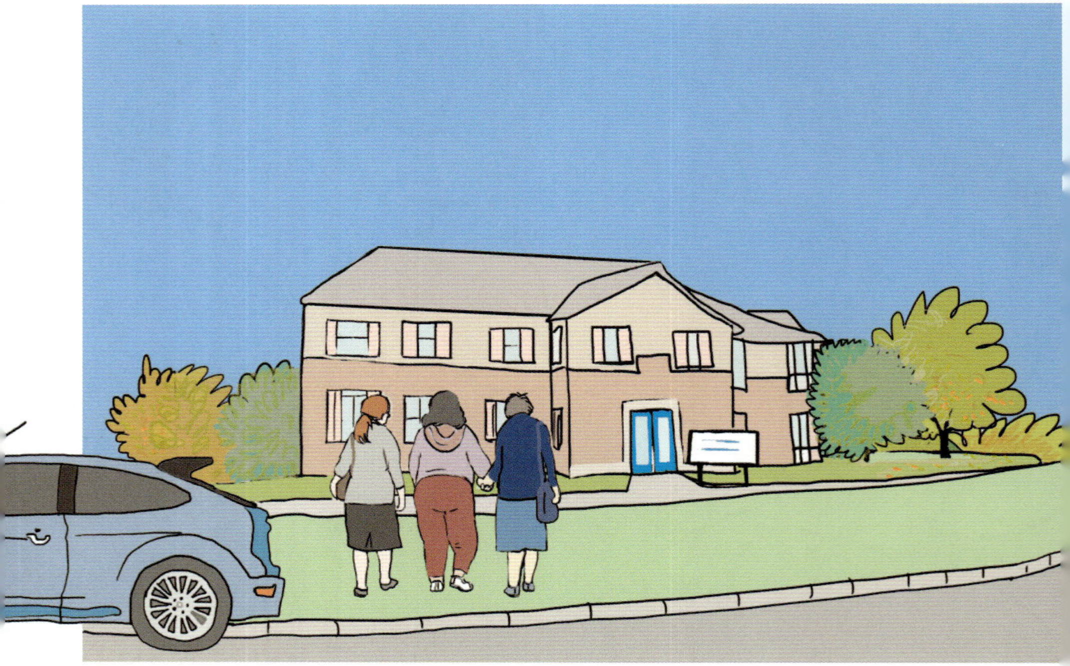

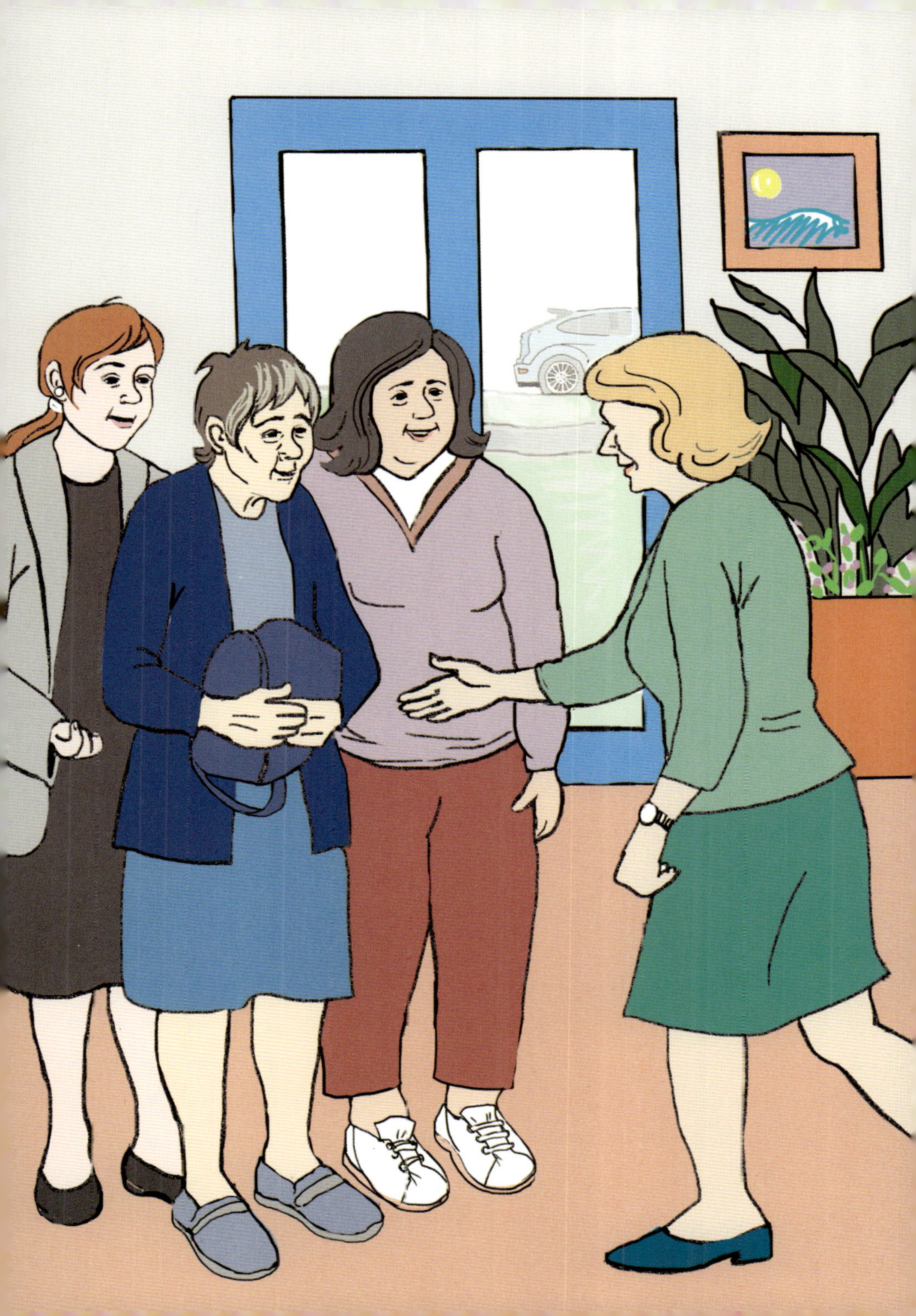

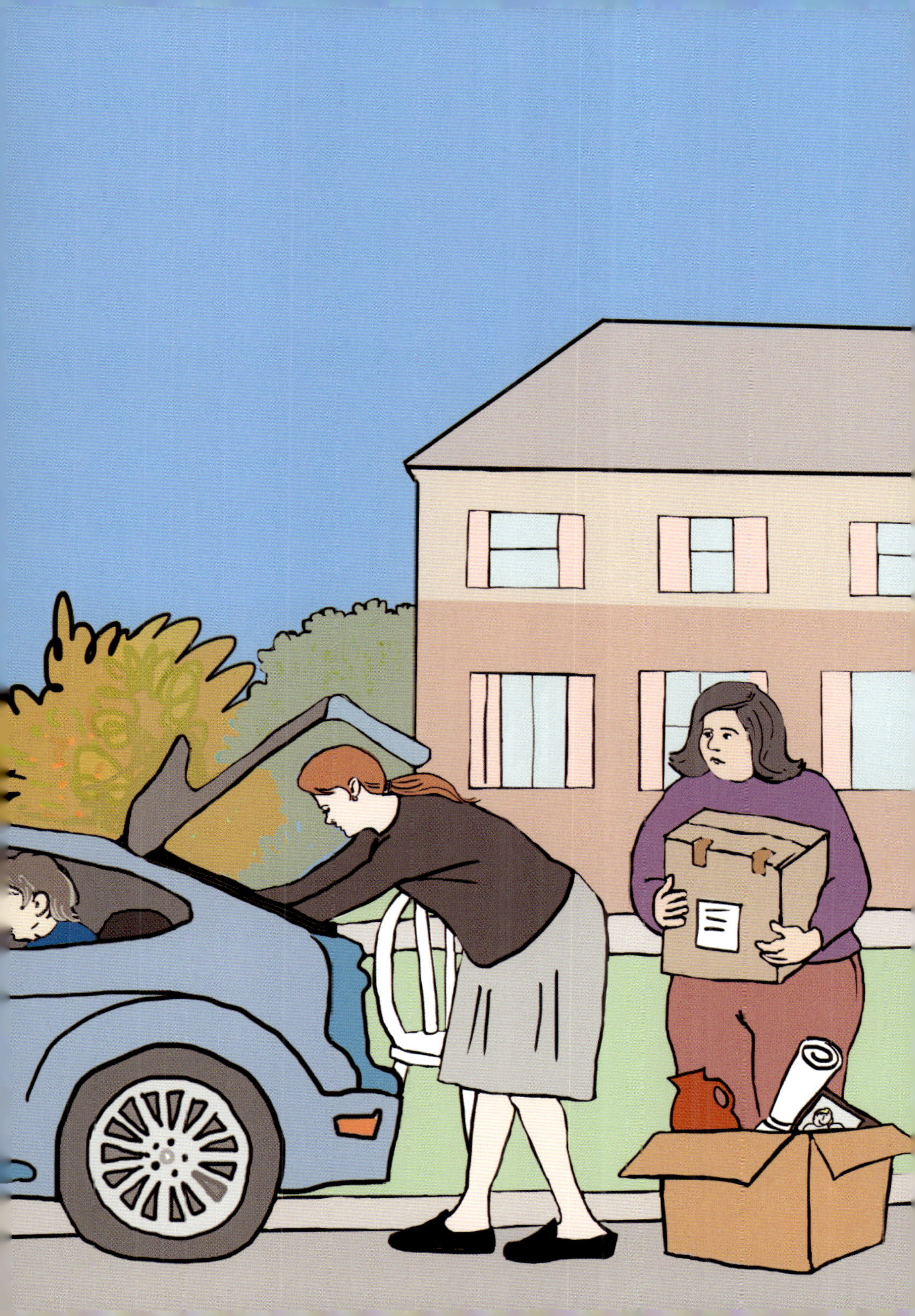

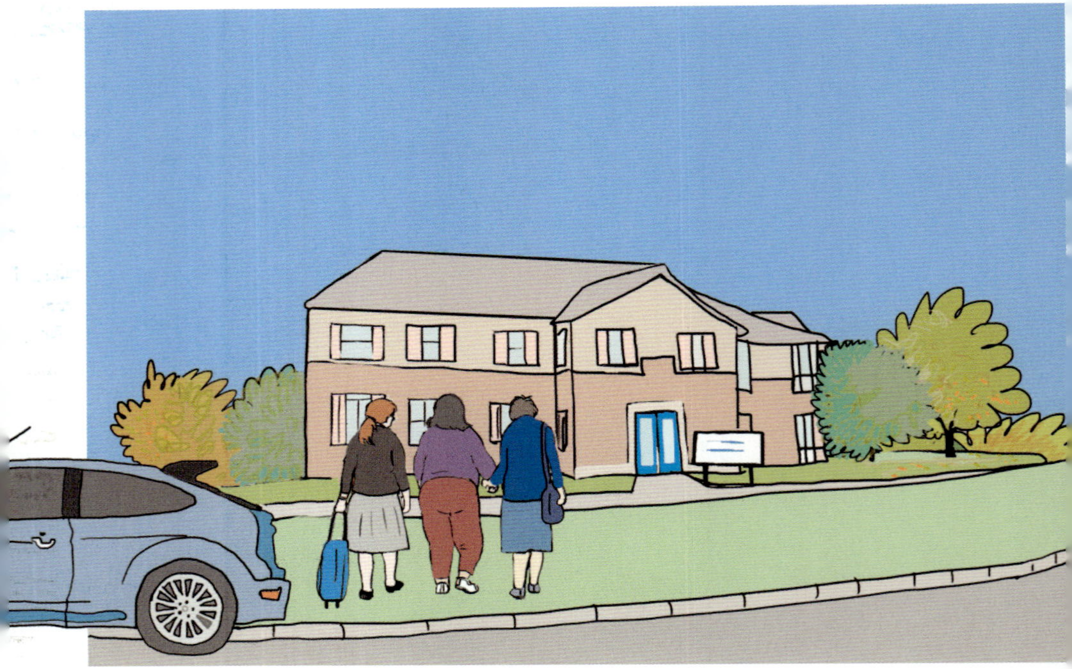

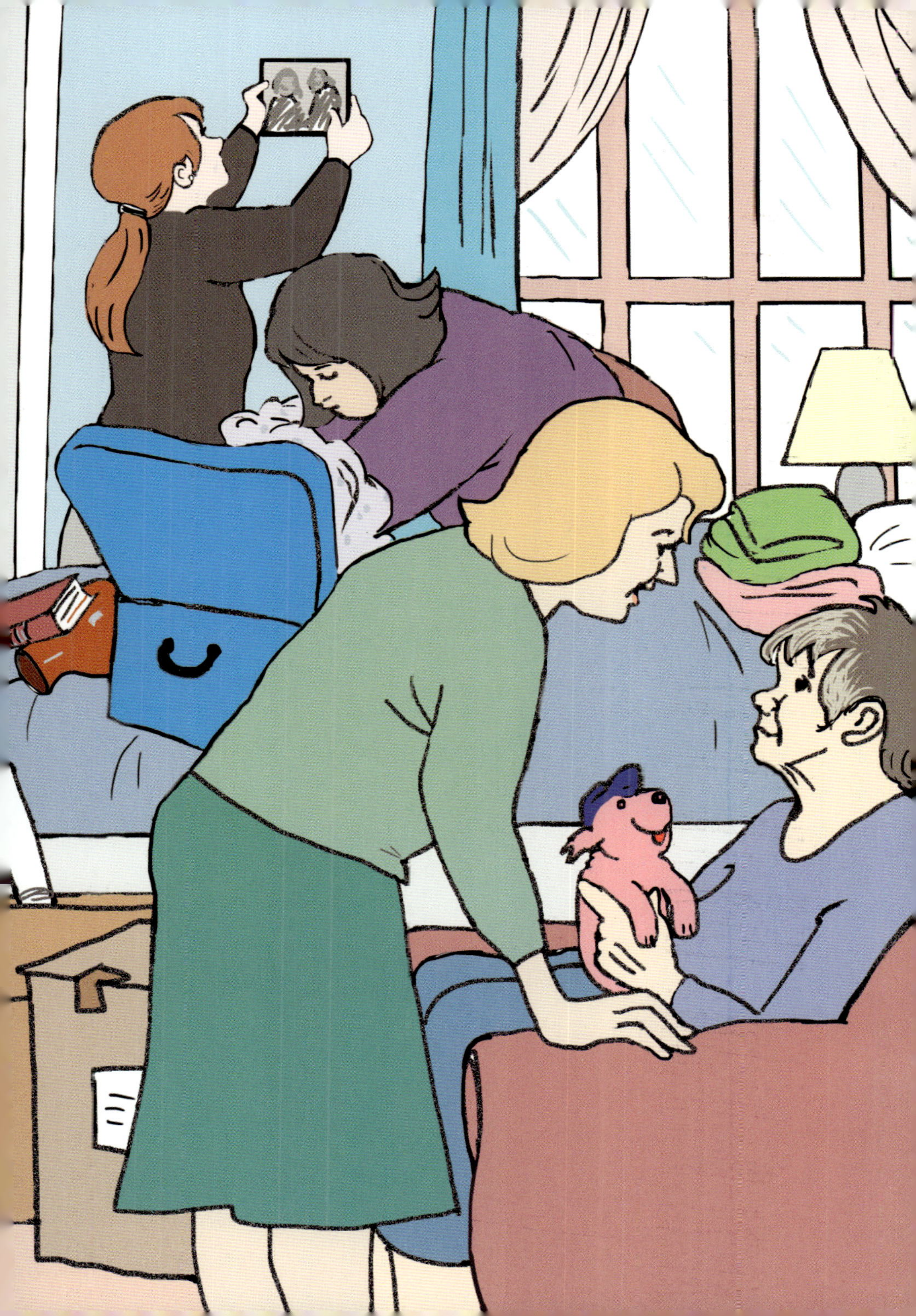

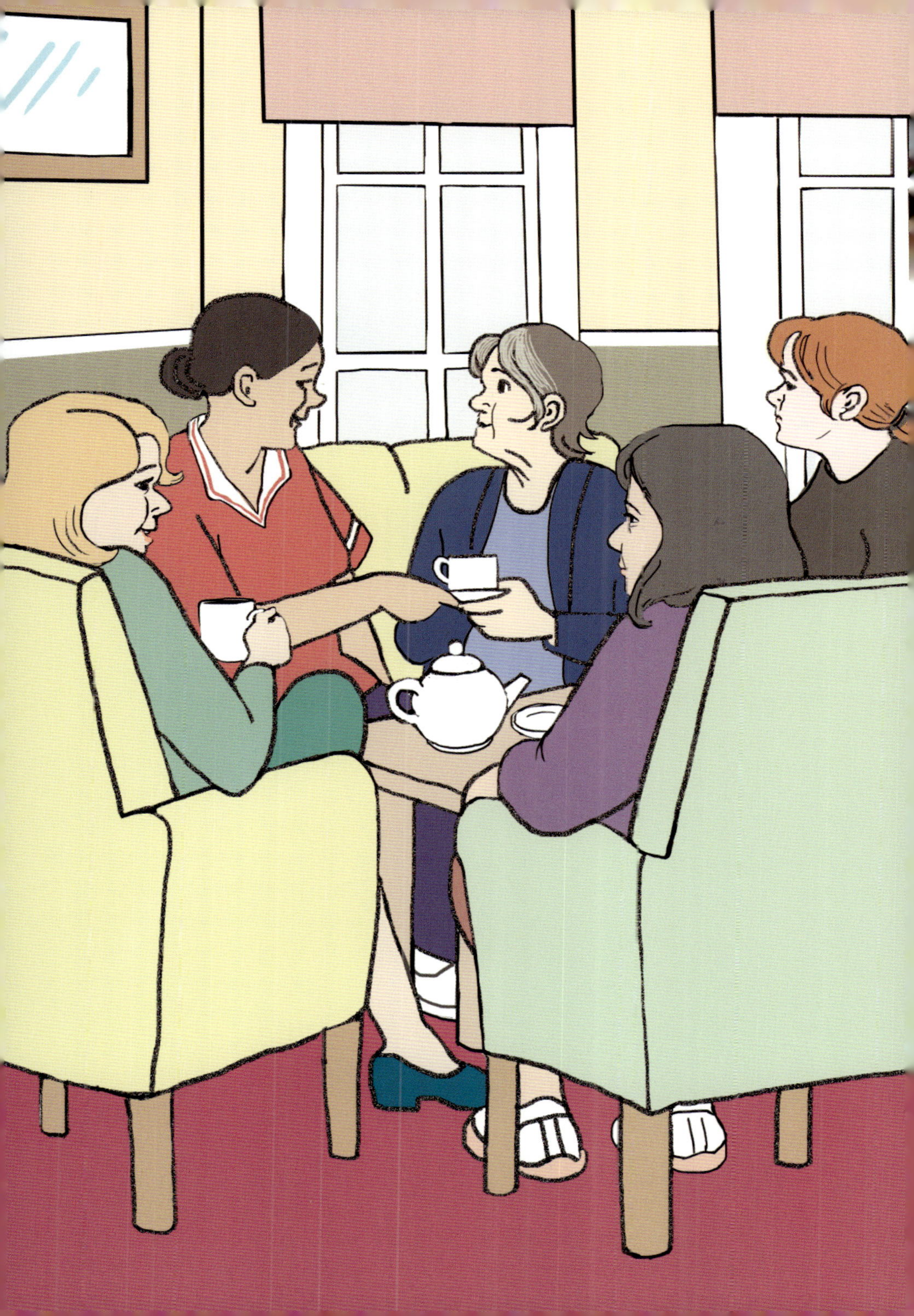

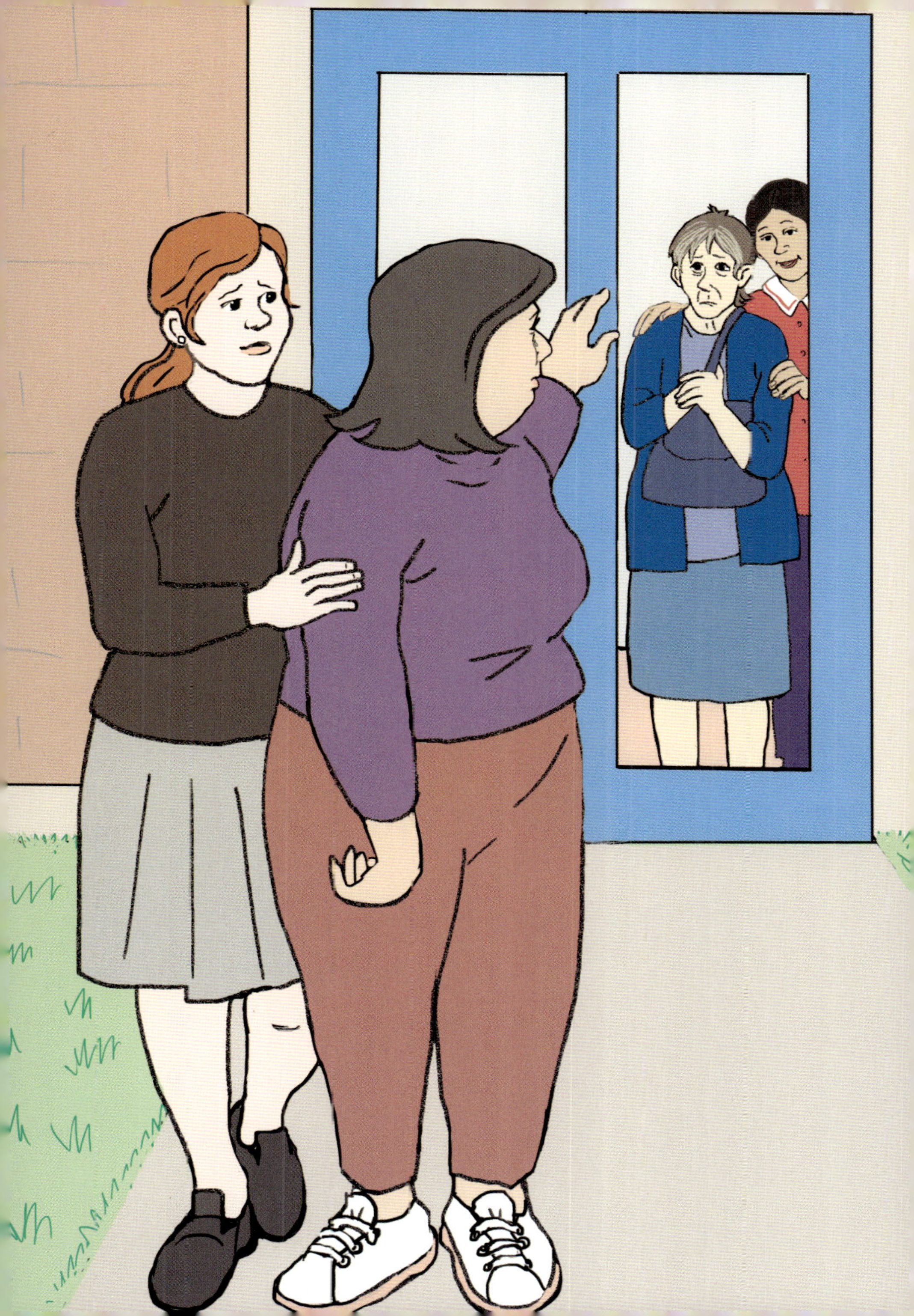

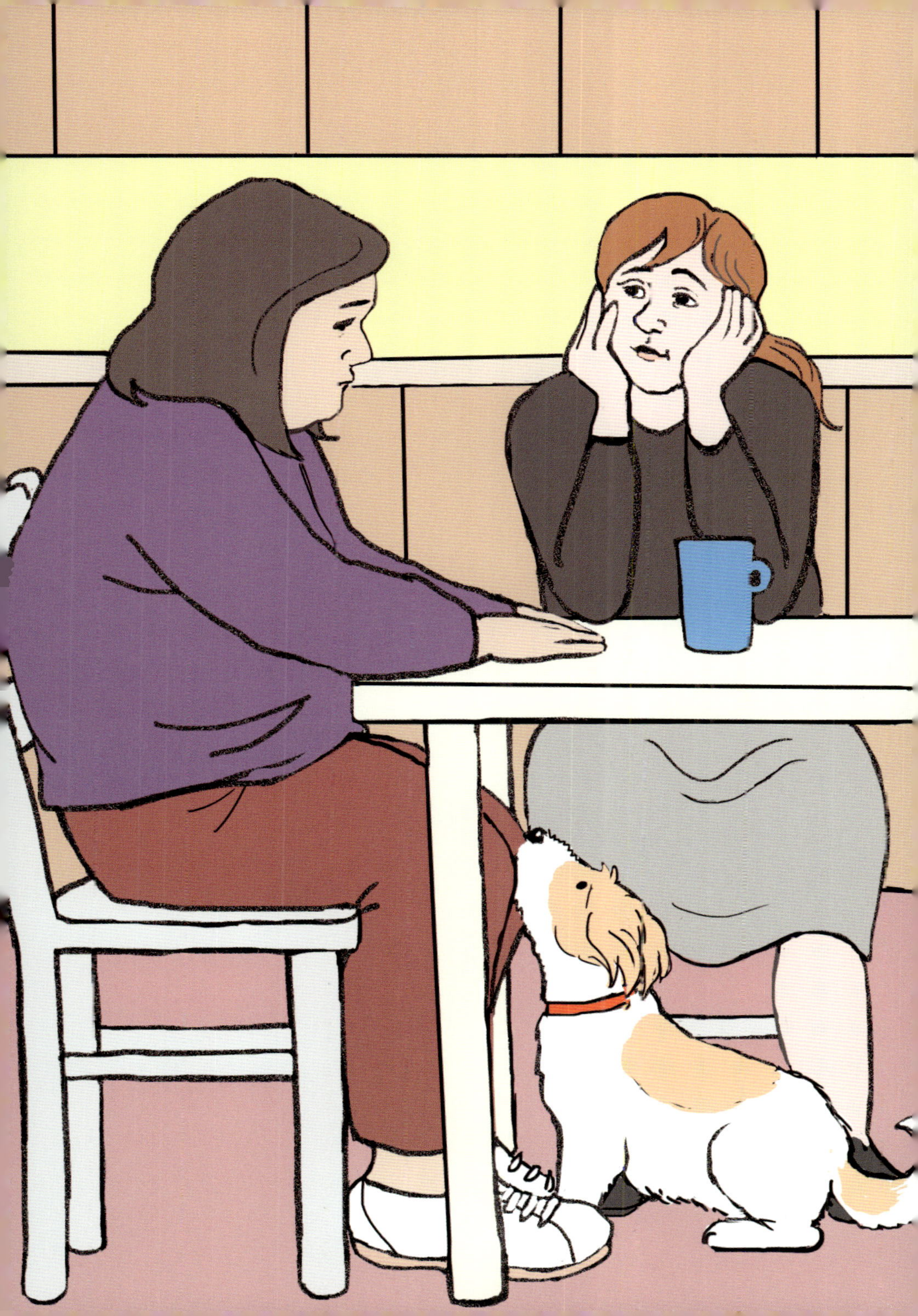

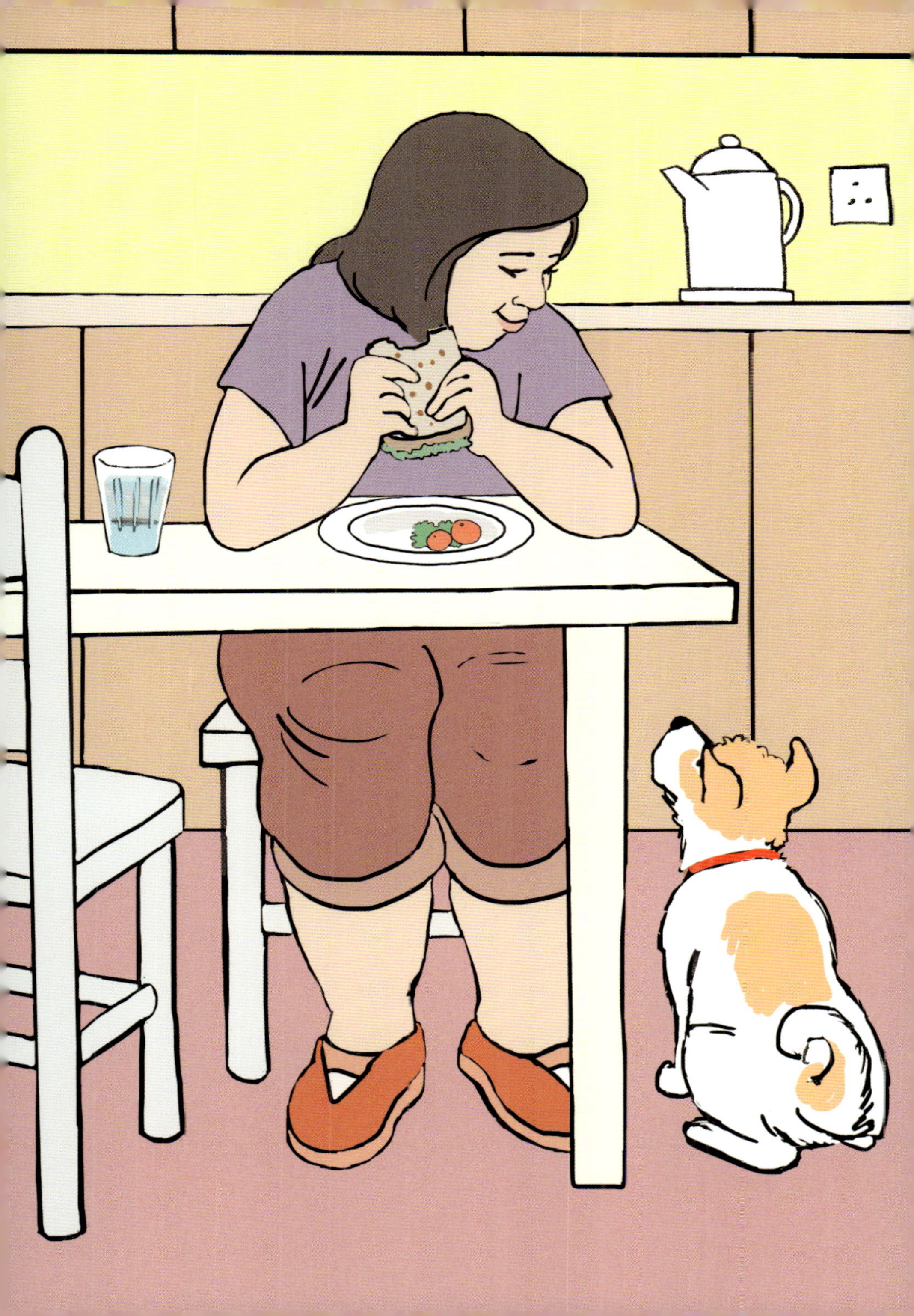

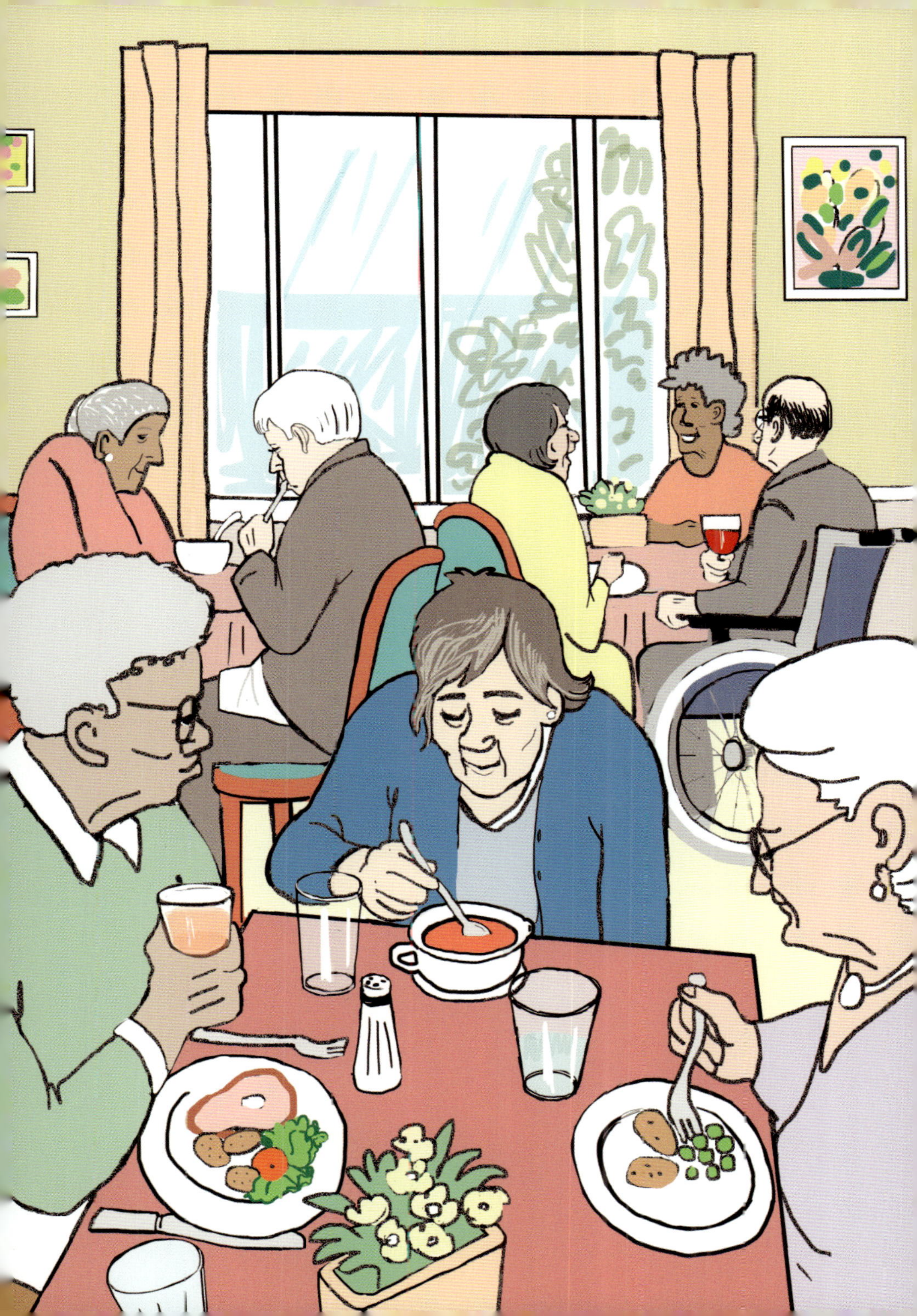

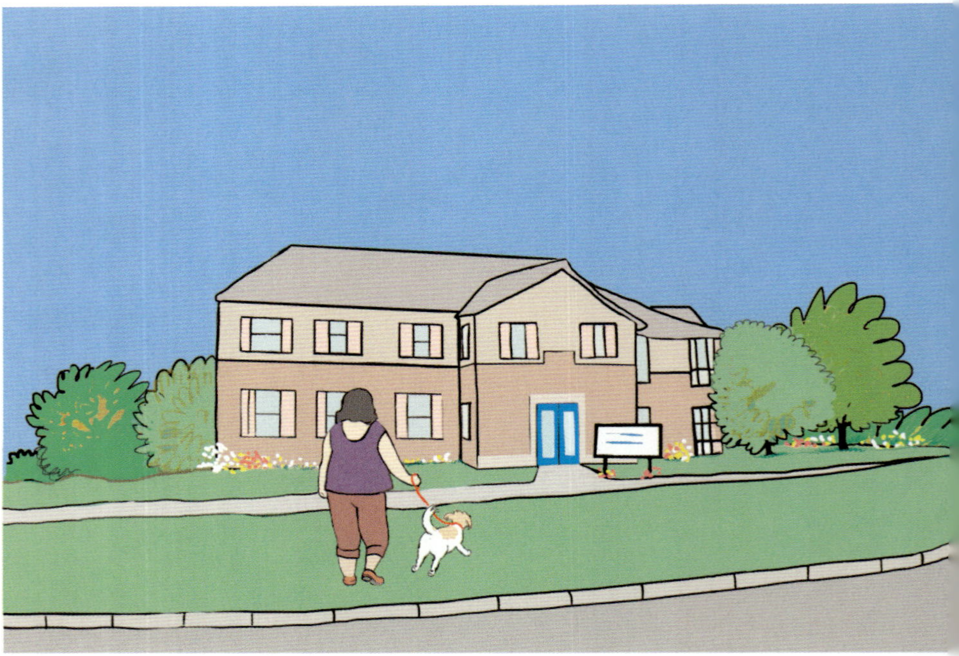

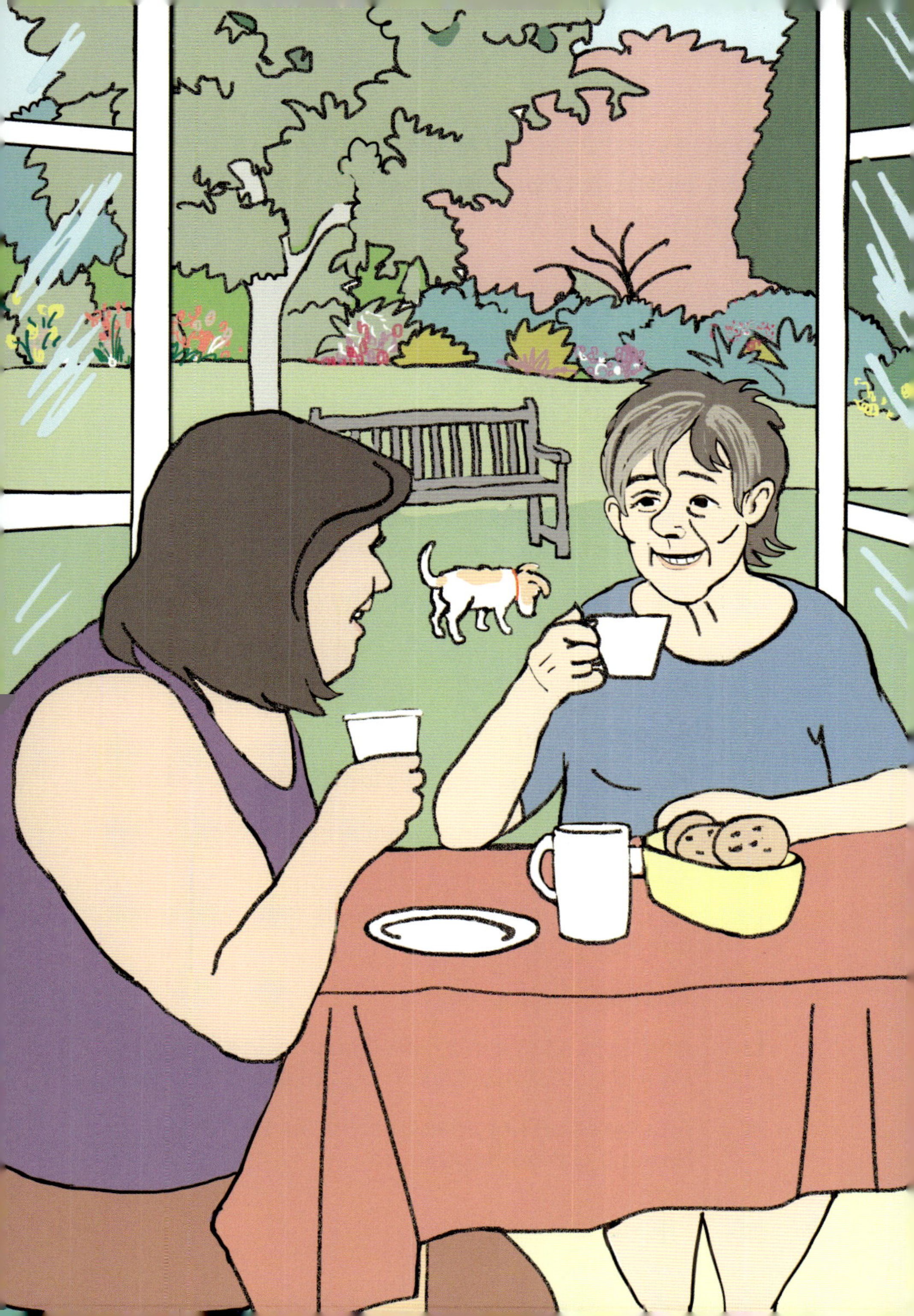

Suggested storyline for readers or carers who want a ready-made story rather than make up their own

1. Ann and Ellen are walking with Goldie, their dog.
2. Ann looks for her key. She can't find it.
3. Oh good! Their neighbour Jo is in. He has a spare key.
4. Jo opens the door for them.
5. Ann and Ellen laugh about Ann's mistake. They have something to drink. The key was at home!
6. Katy comes to see them. They tell her about it.
7. Katy comes often. Today it's raining when she leaves. Ann and Ellen watch TV together.
8. Ellen wakes up. She slept well.
9. What is Ann doing? She's looking for something.
10. Why is the milk in the washing machine?
11. Ann and Ellen eat breakfast together. Both are very quiet. Both are a bit worried that Ann keeps forgetting things.
12. Time to go shopping.
13. Ann finds a table in a café. She puts the shopping on a chair. Ellen brings mugs of tea.
14. Ann takes off her coat. Ellen looks shocked. Ann has still got her nightie on.

15. Ellen puts Ann's coat on quickly. They both feel so embarrassed. Everyone looks at them.

16. They go straight to the doctor.

17. Ellen explains to the doctor what happened. Poor Ann. She looks embarrassed again.

18. The doctor asks Ann to name some common things, like a key or a watch.

19. He rings Katy and tells her about Ann.

20. Katy comes to visit again.

21. Katy asks Ann and Ellen some questions. She makes some notes.

22. Katy has some pictures of different foods. Ellen sticks them on the fridge and cupboards. It will be easier for Ann to find things.

23. Katy rings the nurse and tells her about Ann.

24. Ellen and Ann enjoy sitting in the garden. They play with Goldie.

25. The nurse comes to visit. It's evening time.

26. She helps Ann go upstairs.

27. She helps Ann to have a shower.

28. The nurse helps Ann to go to bed. Ellen and Goldie have come to say good night.

29. Ellen watches TV on her own. She looks relaxed.

30. But why is the front door open?

31. Oh no! Where is Ann? She is not in her bed!

32. Ellen looks out of the window. She can't see Ann anywhere.

33. At last a policewoman brings Ann home. She must be cold in her nightie, with no shoes on.

34. Katy comes with Ann and Ellen to see the doctor. Everyone is worried. How can they keep Ann safe at home?

35. Katy shows Ann and Ellen some photos of different care homes. She asks Ann if she wants to visit one of the homes.

36. Ann and Ellen choose a home to visit. The manager meets them.

37 Soon Ann moves to the new home.

38. Everyone helps to make Ann's new bedroom feel like home.

39. Then they relax in the sitting room. The staff are friendly.

40. Ann and Ellen are both sad when they say goodbye.

41. Katy and Ellen talk about Ann. Ellen feels lost without Ann. Ellen can always talk to Katy about how she feels.

42. Ellen eats on her own. Goldie wonders where Ann is now.

43. Ann eats with other residents in her new home.

44. Ellen visits Ann regularly. Goldie comes too and explores the garden.

Introduction

Just like the rest of the population, people with learning disabilities are living longer. So there are several ways in which they could be affected by dementia. They may have friends or family members who develop dementia or they may develop dementia themselves. This book has been written in such a way that the person in the story who has dementia could be the person with learning disabilities themselves or a family member or friend of the person with learning disabilities. We have left it open so that the story can become whatever is needed for the person who is using the book.

Discussing what they see happening in this book with someone else may help the person to make sense of what is happening in their own life.

When a friend or family member has dementia

It is worrying when someone you know well begins to act strangely, or becomes forgetful or muddled about things. If no one tells you what is wrong, this can be very confusing and can even make you feel cross. It is reassuring to be properly informed about what is happening. The person with dementia will have additional needs which require more attention. It is important that anyone sharing their home does not have their own needs overlooked.

When a person with learning disabilities develops dementia

Not all people with learning disabilities will get dementia. However, people with Down's syndrome are particularly vulnerable. People with learning disabilities who do develop dementia are likely to do so at an earlier age than other people (about 10 years earlier). For those with Down's syndrome this will be even earlier; the average age is 54 years, although it could be as young as 30 years.

The diagnosis can be harder to make in people with learning disabilities and often comes at a later stage of the illness than for other people. This can mean that the time from diagnosis to death will be shorter. For people with Down's syndrome the progression to end-stage dementia is much quicker than for the rest of the population.

Early signs of dementia

It is important to be aware of these possible signs and symptoms and to act on them:

- the person's behaviour may change
- they may seem confused or disorientated
- they may develop memory problems
- there may be changes in their communication
- they may seem more dependent on their senses
- they may have marked changes in their mood or personality
- they may express pain or discomfort through a change in behaviour
- they may seem more susceptible to stress
- they may seem preoccupied
- their sleep patterns may change
- they may be anxious about going out

- they may become confused and wander off
- there may be a deterioration in their abilities
- they may have difficulty in perceiving depth, such as going up a kerb or changing from one surface to another.

If there is any concern, it is important to see a doctor as soon as possible so that the symptoms can be checked out. It is crucial to rule out all other possibilities and to get a clear diagnosis.

Why early diagnosis is important

Getting a diagnosis as early as possible in the illness is important for everyone who has dementia, including people with learning disabilities. It helps all concerned to understand the reasons for the changes in their behaviour or other signs and symptoms, and to work out what help and support are needed. It also enab es the person concerned and their families to think about what help they might need in the future and to make plans accordingly. In the story, Ellen takes Ann straight round to the doctor's when she realises something is very wrong.

How to get a diagnosis

As with everyone else, the first point of contact should be the person's GP, who will discuss their concerns and decide with the individual and their family the best way to obtain an assessment and diagnosis. The usual referral route is to a memory assessment service or memory clinic. Many people with learning disabilities may already be receiving support from a community learning disability team or other secondary service, and so this may be where the best expertise is located and therefore the most appropriate service to undertake the assessment. Many community teams have a nurse or other professional who specialises in dementia and who can offer advice at an early stage.

Identity

Our identity is what makes us unique, being built upon our past and expressed in our present. For people with learning disabilities their shared memories and records of life are easily lost, and when they develop dementia this is even more likely. If they have not already done it, life story work can be a useful tool to maintain the identity of a person with dementia. After diagnosis is not too late to help an individual to put together their life story. This can be in any format that suits that person best – photos, tapes, film clips, writing down their words. It is a way of capturing the things and people that have been and remain important to them in their life. As well as helping the person reminisce about their life, a life story book is a powerful way of bringing the person to life for staff now working with them who may not have known them previously. Further ideas about how to do this can be found at www.lifestorynetwork.org.uk.

Baseline assessments

It can be difficult to recognise the signs of dementia in anyone and perhaps especially in people with learning disabilities. The first step is to establish how the person is when they do not have dementia or when the first suspicions of dementia have occurred. A specialist health professional can carry out a number of tests to establish a baseline of cognitive and other abilities. This then needs to be reviewed regularly by this professional to check on whether and how things change and, if they do, whether there is any sign of dementia. It is important to do this in order that the earliest signs of dementia can be recognised.

Recording signs/changes

The early signs of dementia involve observable change.

- Recording how someone is when they are still healthy establishes a baseline.
- Recording regularly is important.
- Referring back to the baseline allows change to be clearly seen.

Tools such as the CAMDEX (Cambridge Mental Disorders of the Elderly Examination) informant interview and the DisDAT (Disability Distress Assessment Tool) can be helpful.

The recording process is essential in recognising the person's changing needs and how they are experiencing and managing the changes within themselves.

It is important that changes (however small) in all of these areas are recorded in a central file and referred to regularly.

Helping people live well with their dementia

Familiar surroundings and routines and support to maintain interests and abilities are all important for people with dementia. For most people, remaining at home will be what they and their family choose. They may need extra support and adaptations to their home to make this possible. In the early days, this might mean labelling all the rooms and storage spaces clearly to help the person find their way around and find their belongings, as is illustrated in the story. As the illness progresses, the person with dementia may need even more help with their personal care and there may be a need for ramps and handrails or a Zimmer frame.

Family members or the person's support worker can contact their local occupational therapy service for advice. Taking regular exercise, having a healthy diet and continuing to do the things the person enjoys are all helpful strategies. It is also important that everyone around them is calm to avoid unnecessary stress for the person.

It is essential to establish partnerships between everyone involved with the personal care and support of the person with dementia. Each individual holds particular knowledge and understanding of the person.

The following people should be included as appropriate:

- family where possible
- friends
- support workers who know the person well
- GP
- district nurse

- speech and language therapist
- social worker
- residential care manager
- hospital, nursing home or hospice staff
- palliative care team (later on as the illness progresses).

Sharing this knowledge will help in:

- pain management
- medication management
- keeping the person comfortable and safe
- reducing distress.

It is important to try to think about the longer-term needs of the person with dementia. For example, it might be better to support them to change rooms before they become too confused, if it is likely that they will eventually need to have a bedroom downstairs. Ideally, people with dementia should remain in their own home until the end of their life. Their immediate environment should be adapted as their needs change, and the care they receive should be regularly reviewed to make sure it is sufficient.

However, it is possible that the person may not be able to remain at home for a variety of reasons. If a move to residential care becomes necessary, it is important to find ways to make sure that new staff get to know the person as well as they can before they move, and that they have a sense of the person before they had dementia. This is where a life story book is so useful. Familiar and well-loved objects are also helpful; in this story, Ann takes her pink toy dog with her into the home and Ellen visits her with their much loved dog, Goldie.

Useful resources in the UK

Services

Community Learning Disability Teams (CLDTs)

These are specialist multidisciplinary health and social care teams that support adults with learning disabilities and their families by assessment, by supporting access to mainstream healthcare, and by providing a range of clinical interventions. Your GP or Social Services department should have the address of the local team.

Alzheimer's Society
www.alzheimers.org.uk

Provides information, fact sheets and resources about dementia, as well as information on local services that are available nationwide. It also has a national dementia helpline providing information, support and guidance. Tel. 0845 300 0336, usually open from Monday to Friday between 8.30 am and 6.30 pm.

Down's Syndrome Association
www.downs-syndrome.org.uk

Publishes books and fact sheets about Down's syndrome and dementia. Contact their information helpline on 0845 230 0372, from Monday to Friday between 10.00 am and 4.00 pm, to find out about their local support groups.

Training packs, books and DVDs

Dementia and People with Learning Disabilities – Valuing Relationships. By Noëlle Blackman and Michelle Brooks. Designed by Respond and the GOLD Group (a group of older people with learning disabilities). This training pack and DVD is about relationships for people with learning disabilities who develop dementia. You can buy it from www.respond.co.uk/shop.

Down's Syndrome and Dementia Workbook for Staff. By Karen Dodd, Diana Kerr and Scott Fern. For support staff working with people with Down's syndrome who have dementia, enabling them to offer the most effective care possible as the person's condition progresses. It can be bought online from www.downs-syndrome.org.uk.

Food for Thought: A Guide for Supporting People with Down's Syndrome at Mealtimes. A fact sheet about diet and dementia for relatives and carers. Available from Down's Syndrome Scotland (www.dsscotland.org.uk/resources/shop).

In the Know: Implementing Good Practice. By Diane Kerr and Heather Wilkinson. Contains a series of easily accessible, practical and realistic guidance to be used by anyone supporting someone with learning disabilities and dementia. Published by Pavilion Publishing (www.pavpub.com).

Let's Talk about Getting Older. By Lou Marsden. A booklet about getting older for people with learning disabilities. Available from Down's Syndrome Scotland (www.dsscotland.org.uk/resources/shop).

Life Story Network
www.lifestorynetwork.org.uk
Useful resources, an online network and a discussion forum (see the paragraph about identity on page 52).

Related Books Beyond Words titles

Sonia's Feeling Sad (2011) by Sheila Hollins and Roger Banks, illustrated by Lisa Kopper. Sonia is feeling so sad that she shuts herself off from her family and friends. She agrees to see a counsellor and gradually begins to feel better.

Ron's Feeling Blue (2011, 2nd edition) by Sheila Hollins, Roger Banks and Jenny Curran, illustrated by Beth Webb. When Ron retires to bed and shuns his friends, his GP arranges to see him regularly. She helps Ron to enjoy life again.

Am I Going to Die? (2009) by Sheila Hollins and Irene Tuffrey-Wijne, illustrated by Lisa Kopper. This story deals honestly and movingly with the physical and emotional aspects of dying.

When Somebody Dies (2003) by Sheila Hollins, Sandra Dowling and Noëlle Blackman, illustrated by Catherine Brighton. Mary and John are both upset when someone they love dies. They learn to feel less sad by attending regular bereavement counselling sessions and from the comfort and companionship of friends.

When Mum Died and **When Dad Died** (both 2004, 3rd edition) by Sheila Hollins and Lester Sireling, illustrated by Beth Webb. Both books take an honest and straightforward approach to death and grief in the family.

Authors and artist

Sheila Hollins, editor of the Books Beyond Words series, is Emeritus Professor of Psychiatry of Learning Disability at St George's, University of London, and sits in the House of Lords. She is a past President and an Honorary Fellow of the Royal College of Psychiatrists.

Noëlle Blackman is Deputy CEO of Respond, a charity which provides psychotherapy to people with learning disabilities who have experienced abuse or trauma. She has co-facilitated the GOLD group since 1998.

Ruth Eley is an independent health and social care consultant and the former National Programme Lead for older people and dementia in the Department of Health. She is a social worker by training.

Lisa Kopper is a distinguished artist and illustrator of children's books. She is well known for her clear style and ability to draw feelings as well as form, and has illustrated several books in the series.

Acknowledgments

We thank our editorial advisors Paul Adeline and members of the GOLD (Getting Older with Learning Disabilities) Group at Respond for their ideas and advice about what was needed in the pictures: Roger Brooksby, Michael and Sylvia Brookstein, Pat Charlesworth, John Phillips, Sylv Hibbert and Betty Steingold.

We are grateful for the advice and support of our advisory group: Sabyasachi Baumik, Michelle Brooks, Sarah Campbell, Karen Dodd, Peggy Frey, Diana Kerr, Asim Naeem, Satajit Saha, David Thompson, Karen Watchman and Heather Wilkinson.

Finally, we are very grateful to the National Dementia Strategy: Older People and Dementia Team at the Department of Health for providing financial support for this book.

Beyond Words: publications and training

For anyone who wants to help people with learning disabilities to understand their world, including family carers, support workers and professionals.

A list of all **Beyond Words** publications, including **Books Beyond Words** titles, and where to buy them, can be found on our website:

www.booksbeyondwords.co.uk

e-mail: admin@booksbeyondwords.co.uk

Books Beyond Words are also available from: www.amazon.co.uk, and www.amazon.us.com

Workshops on **How to Use Books Beyond Words** are provided regularly in London, or can be arranged in other localities on request. For information about forthcoming workshops see our website. Self-advocates are welcome.

Video clips showing our books being read are also on our website and YouTube channel: www.youtube.com/user/booksbeyondwords, and on our DVD, **How to Use Books Beyond Words**.